EATING
IN THE AGE OF
DIETING

RUJUTA DIWEKAR

EATING IN THE AGE OF DIETING

First published by Westland Publications Private Limited in 2020

Published by Westland Books, a division of Nasadiya Technologies Private Limited, in 2022

No. 269/2B, First Floor, 'Irai Arul', Vimalraj Street, Nethaji Nagar, Alapakkam Main Road, Maduravoyal, Chennai 600095

Westland and the Westland logo are the trademarks of Nasadiya Technologies Private Limited, or its affiliates.

ISBN: 9789395073059

10 9 8 7 6 5 4

Typeset by SÜRYA, New Delhi

Printed at Thomson Press (India) Ltd

CONTENTS

INTRODUCTION

This is how the Upanishads define food—Adyate iti cha bhootani, tasmad annam tad uchayate. That which you consume and in turn consumes you is called as anna or food. And in my twenty years of work, i have learnt that there couldn't have been a better description of the dichotomous, almost paradoxical, relationship that we share with food. The ones who keep it simple and consume it, dare i say, as and when they feel like it, seem to enjoy not just a great equation with food but also with people. They come across as happy, productive and usually enjoy great health too.

On a recent drive from Manali to Kullu airport, something about my driver caught my attention. He was drop dead gorgeous for one, but he seemed to carry a sense of calm that is not usual for people of his age. He looked very young, twenty-three, twenty-five max, but he navigated turns and shifted gears like a pro. 'Kitne saal se gaadi chala rahe ho,' i finally asked. 'Bees saal se,' he said. 'Thirty-eight ka hu.' He had heard my actual question, rare again for a man. 'Wow!' i said. 'Bahut experience hai, bahut accha chalate ho.' 'Haan, lekin abhi two saal mein chodd dunga.' 'Why?' i asked. 'Woh dadi kehti hai ki ab bas hogaya.'

His dadi was eight-five years old and single-handedly looked after the family farm. For as long as he could remember, she would get up by 4 a.m., milk the cows, take them to the jungle, work at the farm, collect wood, etc., and hadn't fallen sick a single day of her life. Just a few days back she had told him, 'Ab bas ho gaya.' She was only going to work for the next two years and wanted to slow down a bit on turning eight-seven. That meant that he could drive only for the next two years and then take on the mantle passed down by dadi and look after the farm and the cattle. His dadi, like every Himachali, also drank copious amounts of tea; Himachalis drink 1 kg of tea per person per year, quite ahead of the 822 gm and 800 gm of Karnataka and Rajasthan who take the second and third positions respectively in chai consumption. 'Aap agar pila do toh dadi fifty-five cups of chai pi legi aur dakaar tak nahi legi. Mujhe toh five cups mein hi gastric ho jata hai,' he said with remorse.

Wow! i really wanted to meet this woman. Because she is not the kind of person that i usually meet. Mostly, i meet people who are at the other end of the spectrum, the ones consumed by food. But since i wrote *Don't Lose Your Mind, Lose Your Weight* in 2009, even the pattern in which we are consumed by food has changed. If earlier it was about intellectualising it, giving it a name or a number (carb, protein, fat, calories, etc.), in the hope to understand it better or eat better or get healthier, now it is about spiritualising it too. 'A cultural appropriation by the diet industry,' as my partner GP calls these new-age diet trends.

The weight-loss industry knows that it is the era of empty rhetoric and it's no longer good enough for a diet to be just a diet; it now needs a cultural spin. And needs to be whipped like a lifestyle. And weight loss may well be their first (and only) plug but it now needs to be dressed as stuff that your ancestors did, will free you from diabetes and cancer, will lead to longevity, etc., etc. 'Ek nur aadmi, sau nur kapda,' goes an old saying in Hindi. It means that a person is only taken as seriously as he dresses or that people are taken in more by appearances than the real thing.

ABOUT THIS BOOK

What is it?

It's a bit indulgent to be honest, but then my editor, Deepthi Talwar, is convinced that it will be helpful for you, my readers, and with that hope here it is. A collection of some of my most-liked articles, columns, interviews and social media posts over the last decade. We are hoping that if individually they touched a chord, then as a collection they will serve the purpose of being a storehouse of information that you can access anytime. There are writings on the basics of good health, on diet trends and food myths, on seasonal foods, festival foods, foods for common health conditions like diabetes, PCOD, etc., home-grown nuskhas for good health, on kids' health and on exercise and yoga. There is also an index that will help you quickly access the topic of your choice.

How to use it?

We have collated the writings in four main sections and thirteen sub-sections. For each sub-section, we have selected writings which give an overview of the topic and those which provide practical and easy-to-follow tips and guidelines. This way, you will not only get to know about the various aspects of our health but also have quick take-aways that you can put into practice immediately. So, there is enough material for everyone at home, for any health problems you might be facing, and for every season and festival. We've also added some heritage recipes to put your culinary skills to test. These have been contributed by my mother, Prof. Rekha Diwekar, tried and tested straight from her kitchen.

Acknowledgements

i think this is as good a time as any to thank all the journalists and editors who gave me the opportunity to write for their newspapers/magazines. Also, to all the people who follow me on my social media handles, and take time out not just to read/watch what i put out there but also generously like, comment and share it with their circle.

Honestly, i shouldn't be complaining; in a way it keeps me in business. But truth be told, it's tough to live in my world and not have my heart break at the things people do to squeeze into dresses, shrink in sizes, and just to drop a few kilos. And to watch repeatedly, over the last two decades, the same excruciatingly painful pattern of being convinced that 'this diet' is going to work. 'This diet' was removing ghee, peanuts, coconut in the '90s. 'This diet' was removing rice, breads, pasta in the mid-

2000s. 'This diet' is currently just not eating anything for sixteen–twenty hours in the day. Every 'this diet' is backed heavily by 'science' and has its followers wanting to convert you into a thinner person with the enthusiasm that would put missionaries to shame.

But. This. Diet. Is. Deprivation. Plain and simple. Sometimes deprived of fat, sometimes of carbs, at other times of the joy of eating. All in the name of weight loss. We seem to have forgotten our basics. That we are worthy of food on our plate. That local, seasonal and traditional food is healthy for people, economies and the planet. That common sense is a science with wide applications to real life. That life is beyond apps, hashtags and social media influencers who juice, cleanse and bullet proof their coffees. Listening to the inner voice was always a difficult task, but with the social media noise and monetisation of your insecurities, it's becoming increasingly difficult to remember that you even have a say in all this.

What we should know is that the more we trap ourselves in the obsession of looking a certain way, the more we play into the hands of the weight-loss industry. And then we lose our connect with the most intimate, intrinsic and instinctive part of our lives—food. And we forget that we can actually stay healthy and look stunning when we eat local foods in sync with the season and in tune with our diverse traditions. That festivals bring us together and that food heals old wounds and bonds us into a social structure that is important for our survival and sanity. That foods with local names are nutritious, delicious and a rare delight. That health comes in all sizes, shapes and weight. And that life must not be spent in looking, speaking and eating like we are clones of each other. That in our diversity lies our strength and stability. The book is essentially my advocacy of this very basic fact. That health is not ghulam to weight, just like love is not ghulam to looks or success to money. i hope you will read with joy, that it will educate you and liberate you from the mad rush of weight loss.

Happy reading and happy eating.

Rujuta Diwekar
October 2020
Mumbai

Section One

FOOD IS A BLESSING

“

RUJUTA SAYS...

Food gives life, not calories.

Face your fears, celebrate your efforts, eat without guilt, life is beautiful at every size.

The biggest lie ever been told is that you have to give up on traditional food and cuisine to lose weight.

Fitness is like a relationship; the only way to sustain it is through love, commitment and daily effort.

Only love happens in an instant; diet and exercise take at least twelve weeks to show results.

Eating right is a skill just like swimming and cycling; you may take time to learn it but once you do, it stays with you forever.

”

1A. BASICS OF GOOD HEALTH

Health is happiness

Health is not just about the absence of disease, but rather the presence of enthusiasm and aspiration, an ability to learn at every stage in life. It encourages one to be on—and stay on—a path of happiness and fulfilment.

Let's start with the Upanishads, a collection of texts central to many beliefs of Hinduism, Buddhism and Jainism. The Upanishads describe sukha, or happiness, as a state where our senses—sight, smell, touch, sound and taste—are all aligned with one another. Dukha, on the other hand, is a state where the senses are not aligned and is, naturally, the lack of happiness. Each of us has experienced this: the body in one place, the mind in another and the senses distraught. This lack of alignment is what the modern world calls 'stress'.

In Ayurvedic terms, 'health' can be translated as swasthya, a state where the swa (the self), is stha (centred). In other words, health is synonymous with the state of being centred, with all senses aligned—or as Mahatma Gandhi described it, a confluence of thought, speech and action, and no conflict between them. Yoga, for one, guides us to health on the path of shanti, or peace, and the yoga texts teach us that swasthya is step one to both inner and outer peace.

Satvik food is simple, sensible and seasonal

1. **Simple**: Food which is cooked at home, which you have grown up eating, which your grandmother recognises. E.g. Dal-chawal-ghee for dinner and not soups and salads.
2. **Sensible:** Eating food with common sense and with all senses, counting prana instead of calories, eating wholesome and not in parts, and eating fresh and not packaged and processed. E.g. Poha, upma, idli, dosa, paratha for breakfast and not packaged cereals and oats.
3. **Seasonal**: Food which is fresh, in season, which grows locally in the same environmental conditions, and also food according to the season. E.g. Jowar in summer and bajra in winter instead of multigrain bread.

Eat local, think global

The world today is fatter than what it was just ten years ago, and yet the dangers of hunger loom over us just as much as they did. Globally, we are facing what is called as the double burden of malnourishment. On the one hand is a population that eats so much that they could die because of the excesses, and on the other hand is a population that doesn't have access to three square meals a day.

This issue surely deserves the attention of governments, needs serious policy changes and more importantly advocacy for local food and food systems. And this is where each one of us can contribute individually. As a regular traveller, you must have noticed that from Kashmir to Kanyakumari, Bangalore to Boston, every airport serves the same food from the same big food chains. The burger, the pizza, the coffee chains dominate, and even after a long hunt, a restaurant that serves local food or even a local beverage is hard to come by. And it's exactly this uniformity in eating across the globe post the industrialisation period that is the leading cause of obesity, and now, as scientists are beginning to realise, of climate change too.

Local food is climate resilient. It blends into the local food systems and grows in a manner that allows for other crops and the surrounding eco-system of fruits, flowers, insects, bees, etc., to flourish. It's nutrient rich and, by default, a culture fit for the population of that land. It makes economic sense too, as it allows small farmers to grow local food without heavy investments (and unpredictable returns) into bio-technology, modified seeds and even labour. All in all, it helps keep the people, their land and their forest in a good shape.

Essentially, it's about going back to the wisdom of our forefathers, of eating local, regional and seasonal. What it needs is the glam quotient. Local food is where yoga was twenty-five years ago—waiting to be adopted, valued and packaged as the healthiest thing you could be on.

THE SELF-LIMITING CURVE

i was recently invited to Jordan to speak about yogic wisdom on eating right and how eating according to traditional Indian food wisdom leads to a lean body and a meditative mind. Eating what is local, fresh and seasonal, eating slowly and learning to stop before the stomach is stuffed is an integral aspect of leading a yogic lifestyle.

It's also based on the common sense that only the person who digests the food should decide how much to eat, not some dietitian. Learning to eat till one feels light and energetic and not dull and torpid needs practice. Appetite is a moving entity and we are all differently hungry, and that's exactly why diets which reduce humans to a set of numbers—height, weight, calories—invariably backfire.

Arab culture has a beautiful system in place, one that is in tune with the yogic philosophy of eating light and right. You are only allowed either one, three, five, seven—basically an odd number of cups—for Arabian coffee with dates, both local to the region. This has an inbuilt system to respect the fact that the human stomach has different needs every day and ensures that you don't land up over-eating/drinking. On a day you feel like two cups of coffee, you stop at one, on a day you are feeling like four you stop at three, at all times leaving part of the stomach empty. It allows for easy movement of food within the stomach and leaves you feeling light in the body and meditative in the mind.

The world's healthiest diet

If you asked me what the world's healthiest diet is, i would say it is the one that keeps you connected with: 1. Farms 2. Forests and 3. Family heritage.

Because then it would allow you to view vegetables like aloo or colocasia in good light. Then you would value it for being the wild and uncultivated vegetable of the monsoon. You would pay a farmer who didn't have to invest heavily in labour or chemicals to grow it. Your family would have at least three recipes to cook it. And you would have friends who would devour it.

All of this is important because food plays higher roles in our lives than what we realise. It brings people together, it teaches us to eat in sync with the climate, it allows us to develop gratitude for those who grow and cook our food.

And in increasingly lonely lives full of free wi-fi and unlimited diet fads, we should hold on to that connect with our food like our life depends on it, because it really does depend on it.

The three pillars of good health

Food | Exercise | Sleep

1. *Food*

Local | Seasonal | Traditional (cooking/recipes)

Local and seasonal produce will provide all the nutrients you need and traditional methods of cooking will ensure that these nutrients are available for your body to assimilate.

2. *Exercise*

Strength | Flexibility | Stamina

Your workouts should address all these parameters and not focus on just one of these. Also, at least 150 minutes of exercise every week should be the goal.

3. *Sleep*

Two- to three-hour gap after dinner | No gadgets sixty to ninety minutes prior | Fixed bedtime and wake-up time

Good sleep is crucial to ensure that you recover from exercise and that the food you ate can give you the nutrition you need. Also, plays a big role in hormonal balance.

Health professionals

A good doctor:

1. Instils confidence, not fear.
2. Cares about understanding your history beyond blood tests.
3. Develops a vocabulary to explain why what you have read on Google may/may not be relevant to your case (no rhetoric like 'doctor kaun hai?').
4. Keeps your time, as emergencies are not a daily affair (especially if it's not a government hospital/clinic).
5. Doesn't tell you to lose weight, but instead asks you to get fitter, stronger and exercise.

A good dietitian:

1. Gives you food-based and not nutrient-based guidelines.
2. Teaches you about food systems and not food groups.
3. Plans meals that are suitable to culture, community, region. Stays away from dos and don'ts list.

4. Encourages exercise and understands that walking is an activity, not exercise.
5. Sets you on the path of getting progressively fitter and not fatter. Junks the weighing scales.

A good trainer:
1. Teaches you to pursue fitness and not thinness.
2. Tweaks the dose of exercise based on your ability to recover from it.
3. Trains you for strength, stamina, mobility, flexibility and not for weight loss.
4. Educates you about muscles, movements, machines and not about the latest affair in the gym.
5. Looks out for you and not for phone notifications.

When the latest in nutrition science catches up with dadis and nanis

Highlights of Canada food guide, 2019

- Nutritious food can reflect cultural preferences and traditions.
- Eating together brings enjoyment, and fosters relationships between generations and cultures.
- Traditional food improves the quality of your diet.

What's more?

- Stresses on the importance of eating local.
- Recommends eating more protein from pulses and legumes (not just meat).
- Emphasises thinking about the environmental impact of your food choices.
- Most importantly, gives NO PORTION SIZES; instead tells you to pay attention to hunger and satiety.

Basically, never trade common sense for science, because science eventually catches up. And say thank you to your grandmom, look at her with renewed respect; being ahead of her times was her only crime.

Count what matters

Instead of body weight—the number of meals you eat outside or from packets.
Instead of body fat percentage—the number of workouts you do every week.
Instead of heart rate—how energetic or tired you feel.
Instead of sleep timers—how clear the skin looks or constipation or bowel movements.
Instead of the number of steps—the number of times you felt a sugar craving in the week.

Apps don't inform, they target you for your vulnerabilities. Health comes with taking responsibility for the self and not delegating it to an app.

App or Appa?

Food as a number	**Food as a blessing**
Eat a fixed portion	Eat as per appetite
Obsessed with food	Celebrate life beyond the body
Focus on results	Focus on the journey
Cheating during festivals	Celebrations during festivals

Food as a number	Food as a blessing
Customised to carbs, proteins, fats	Customised to culture, cuisine, climate
Exercise as punishment/ compensation	Exercise as an integral part of life

Servings of self-empowerment

'Eat rice? Cool. But you'll tell me how much i can eat, right? Should i send my driver to fetch my plate and katori?' asks my client.

'i don't need to know the size of your katori or plate; eat as much as you want,' i tell her. 'How will i lose weight then?' she shoots back, throwing her hands in the air, exasperated. That's it: she is convinced she will never lose weight if she eats as much as she wants.

Have you ever asked anybody how much money you should be making? Just like money, food is a resource too. And just like money, abusing food or investing your calories in the wrong foods has side-effects.

This paranoia with quantity is a modern-day curse that we have brought upon ourselves. The weight-loss industry has us convinced that we are simply incapable of stopping ourselves at the right amount; and that we need somebody, preferably a trained and certified dietitian, to constantly monitor our food portions and reprimand us if we've eaten 'more' than prescribed.

i find this trend ridiculous. If you are listening to anybody other than your stomach for advice on determining quantity, you are doomed to stay fat. Your stomach is your biggest diet guru, and if you are attuned to your gut, you will know the exact quantity you need to set the fat-burning process, well, burning. Eat less than what you need, and you set the stage to overeat at the next meal. Eat too much, and you have already overloaded your stomach.

The key is to eat out of need and not greed, or even worse, guilt. It's easy to figure out your needs if you listen to your stomach: the signals are loud and clear. The question is, are you paying attention or are you just changing channels and discussing the latest fad diet that's been cooked up? *(See infographic on page 13)*

The 'eat right' plan

How are you feeling today? Did you sleep well last night? Have you been complying with your exercise plans? Do you have sweet cravings post meals?

How many of us consider the above factors as a reflection of our health? But that's what they are, surrogate measures of metabolic health—your hormonal health, cholesterol levels, kidney and liver functions, gut health and much more. However, the public health narrative is almost always about losing weight. Often, at the cost of health gain.

This is why we started the twelve-week fitness project in the beginning of 2018. It was to reinforce common

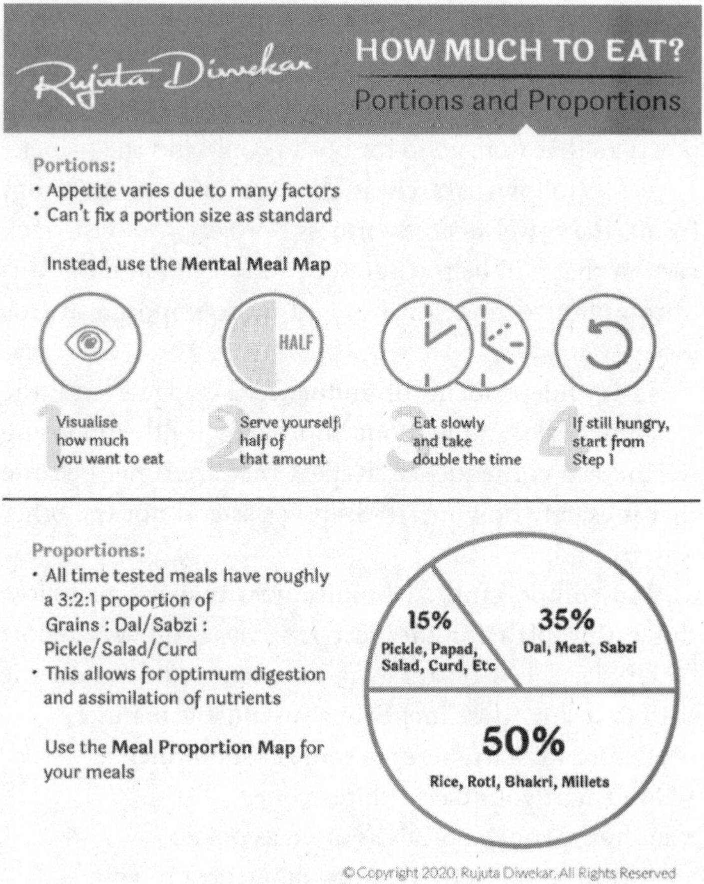

sense and put control back in the individual's hands as far as health goes. More than 1.25 lakh people from over forty countries participated and saw improvements in metabolic health parameters, inch loss from their waists and developed a better relationship with food.

Most importantly, the culturally compliant food and lifestyle modifications were sustainable, as most participants continued following them. Fitness doesn't have to cost you the earth, literally. It's 2020, climate change is a reality, and we need to go back to eating practices that were good for both people and the planet.

What follows is a cheat sheet to essential learnings from the twelve-week fitness project, a fast-track version that will help you reset yourself in ten days. It is uncomplicated, inexpensive, and more importantly, it's easy.

It is independent of influencers, gadgets and the weighing scale, and is about improving health and losing weight as a consequence. Repeat that after me. Because that is exactly how metabolism works and not the other way around.

Most importantly, i promise you that if you follow this eating plan for the next ten days, you will report better sleep, less bloating, more energy, and be on the path to losing those inches in a sustainable manner.

Before we start, here are some ground rules:

- Don't start your day with tea/coffee.
- Eat home-cooked meals as often as possible.
- Eat your meals without your phone next to you.
- Structure your meals as follows: pre-breakfast, breakfast, mid-morning snack, lunch, 4–6 p.m. meal, dinner.
- Patronise what grows around you, is in season and is cooked in your kitchen.

Meal plan

1. *Eat a banana or any other fresh fruit first thing in the morning.* Or soaked almonds or soaked raisins. You

can have a traditional home-cooked breakfast (idli, dosa, poha) about forty-five minutes to an hour after this.

Why: Fitness is built one step at a time by small but daily actions. The body rewards consistency over anything else.

2. *Add ghee to every meal—do this gradually if this is a new habit.* So, add ghee to one meal first, then gradually increase it. Put in as much as enhances the taste of the food and does not mask it. Also, take into account the food item: rice-dal, roti-vegetable will need lower quantities; puran poli, dal baati will need more.

Why: Ghee is the ultimate Indian superfood. It is a fat that breaks down other fats, is excellent for digestion, keeps joints healthy and skin glowing. Ghee also reduces sweet cravings.

3. *Have a mid-morning snack.* You can have a fresh fruit or a homemade laddoo or barfi (traditionally made as per season). Or a seasonal/homemade drink such as coconut water, buttermilk, nannari, nimbu sherbet (with not more than one teaspoon sugar), etc.

Why: The Ayurvedic wisdom behind including these drinks during the day was to stoke the appetite, ease digestion and boost the immune system. They introduce diversity to your diet, allowing you to celebrate the season, through eating roots, flowers and leaves.

4. *The 4–6 p.m. meal is your most important meal of the day.* Plan this as carefully as you would your lunch or dinner. You could eat a chapatti with ghee and jaggery. Or choose between poha, upma, dosa, egg-toast, murukku or homemade coconut, gram or gond laddoo. If you have early dinners, then just have some groundnuts with jaggery.

Why: i always tell my clients that the key to losing weight lies in what they eat between 4 p.m. and 6 p.m., a time when most of us are very hungry and also the most careless in our eating. By eating something wholesome in the evening, you can eat a light dinner. This is the make-or-break meal; this decides whether you will have long-lasting fitness or whether it will fizzle out in the next couple of weeks.

5. *For dinner, eat rice with sambar, rasam or dal and any vegetable you want to add*. For the rice, pick hand-pounded or single-polished rice, instead of brown rice, for your everyday use.

Why: This is easy to digest, and a complete meal. Rice and dal also improves sleep quality. It is suitable for people of all kinds of constitutions according to Ayurveda (vata, pitta and kapha doshas).

A public appeal

Lockdown has made us fall in love with home-cooked food again. Don't let that go.

The current crisis has forced us to relook at many aspects of our life—be it work, travel or relationships. And it seems to have driven home one point: let's get back to basics. In a sense, it has brought out the romantic in us. People are posting and raving about the blue skies, the sighting and chirping of birds and—this almost brings a lump to my throat—the goodness of dal-rice. It's like people have realised that the most intimate relationship we share is with food, and it remains central to our lives, especially to our quarantine life.

In a sense, it took a pandemic for people to see that food is much more than a sum of carbs, fat and protein. And the macros that matter are safety, survival and sustenance. The panic shopping, even at the risk of getting infected, is a testament to just that. For the first time in the twenty years of my career, i am being asked questions about immunity-boosting foods. Till now it was only about what can one do to accelerate fat-burning. i am enjoying this interest, celebrating it.

It's wonderful to see people return to basics, to discover that when you are short on time and other resources but still need to eat to stay strong and secure, it is the khichdi that comes through, not the smoothie. The question, though, is whether the learnings of the lockdown will stay with us. Will the love for home-cooked food and virtuosity of jhadu-pocha transition into our real lives once things are back to normal?

Well, i am a sceptic. In the early 1990s, when Cuba faced food and fuel shortages due to the US embargo, Cubans took to small-scale gardening and cycling, and as a population lost weight and rates of heart disease and diabetes dropped. But when the economy picked up in the new millennium, those habits didn't stick, and weight and related diseases rose. Long story short, disasters or emergencies may throw up a few good things, but they don't make for a life-long learning. Not when it's forced.

So, once life is back to normal, actively re-initiate your love for home-cooked food. What you are doing right now is a one-night stand, but it's worthy of a long-term relationship. Pursue it once the lockdown is over.

“

RUJUTA SAYS...

To lose weight, eat local and not low-cal. ;-)

Losing weight without eating right and exercising is like marrying without trust and faith.

Wajan nahi negativity kam karo toh bhojh uttar jayega.

If happiness is a prisoner of body weight, it's not happiness, it's hallucination.

You are free to feel happy and worthy at any size and weight. Exercise that freedom.

Weight-loss is not about getting there fast but staying there forever!

”

1B. HEALTH BEYOND WEIGHT LOSS

The business of health

In everyone's life there's always one person who has tried his hand at all kinds of businesses and failed. But the math of failure upturns when you enter the world of weight loss. Almost every person who has tried to lose weight has failed to keep it off. And it's not from a lack of trying. It could actually be a case of trying too much. Statistics put the number of people who have lost weight and kept it off at less than 20 per cent, which means that at least 80 per cent of us are constantly struggling to lose weight. India, by the way, is the third-most obese country in the world.

We also rank amongst the highest in the global hunger index, just behind Afghanistan and Pakistan. This lethal combo of obesity and hunger is described as the double burden of malnourishment by the World Health Organisation. 'Not too long ago in our country, the main difference between the rich and the poor was not the food they ate but the clothes they wore,' said a seventy-year-old farmer from Sangli, part of a senior internship programme in my office. That is clearly changing.

This double burden is a global phenomenon. The number of underweight people has gone up from 330 million in 1975 to 462 million in 2014. But in the same period, we have gotten fatter—a number that stands at 641 million, up from 105 million. For the first time ever, the planet has more obese than underweight people.

The biggest culprit for this change is the rural-to-urban shift in population, which comes with a decrease in physical work and a shift in diet patterns. The cost of living in cities is higher and women stepping out to work has not been accompanied with men leaning in, in kitchens. Gender equality, a determinant for health and wellbeing, is consigned to fantasy life on the big screen, like in *Ki & Ka*.

In reality, the additional income gets diverted into buying more readymade food, essentially food that is poorer in quality of nutrients, but often packaged as healthy. Urban life and open markets have not just meant a Zara next door, but even the import of processed food into daily life. But it doesn't stop here. Globalisation has also meant the importing and blind acceptance of nutritional culture—guidelines, diets, eating habits—from the developed world; all of which adds to the epidemic of obesity hitting our country.

By the 1970s, the West had declared 'fat' as the biggest villain in our diets, arguing it was the main cause of heart disease. India responded by promptly striking ghee off its healthy list. Fast-forward to 2016, and the United States Food and Drug Administration has changed its stand on fat, and more specifically cholesterol, saying that cholesterol 'is a nutrient that is no longer a concern for over-consumption'.

The media has always followed this yo-yo approach. In 1984, the cover of *Time* had an image of eggs and bacon with the headline, 'Cholesterol: And Now the Bad News'. In 1999, the picture was of eggs and a piece of fruit with a caption saying eggs are okay but margarine (hydrogenated vegetable fat made to replace bad butter) was a problem. The 2014 cover had a dollop of butter on it and declared: 'Scientists Labeled Fat the Enemy. Why They Were Wrong'.

Forty years is a long enough time for a fear to spread and for people to change their default 'eat healthy' setting to 'avoid ghee on roti' and other essential fats like makhan on a paratha. The current villain that causes all lifestyle diseases is sugar. It has replaced the position that fat had in the 1970s. Will it return as the champion that helps people avoid lifestyle diseases forty years later? Your guess is as good as mine.

In 2012, the fitness and slimming industry was worth about Rs 6,000 crore and growing at a rate of 20 per cent. The nutrition food, beverages and supplement market crossed Rs 100 crore in 2015. Dry-fryers account for one of the biggest segments of India's electronic market today, while even biscuit advertisements position their products as health snacks, to capture audiences.

Essentially, as the weight-loss market continues to grow, so do the number of diabetics and obese people in our country. It's time we ask ourselves if we're looking for information in the wrong places. Are we interpreting data incorrectly? Is the industry making profits at the cost of keeping us fat?

It all started when we were asked to avoid calories, and in the process of avoiding them, we began to view food from the narrow window of carbs, protein and fats instead of the larger picture of eating local, seasonal and fresh. Nutrition experts across the world are now waking up to the fact that science needs to come out with food-based and not nutrient-based guidelines. At a conference i attended in 2012 in Newcastle, UK, food scientists admitted that breaking up food by its main nutrients like carbs, protein and fat has been counterproductive.

These were meant to allow the average person make informed decisions about food. However, it has only served the interest of weight-loss, food and pharma companies. Depending on the latest villain, the packet that labels itself as 'xxx free'—fat-free in the 1990s, sugar-free in the 2000s and gluten-/dairy-free now—is priced 40 per cent higher than a regular product. So you can buy a packet of chips that's vegan and gluten-free or a soda that's sugar-free and feel happy to pay more for it.

Nutrient-based guidelines have also started the trend of 'expert' endorsements. So you have oils, cereals or yoghurts that are backed by medical or diabetic associations and mirror the latest trend. Vegetable oils like sunflower oil came packaged with an illustrated heart to show that doctors have certified its heart-healthiness. Yet, recent research has shown that traditional local oils—groundnut, sesame, coconut, mustard—are far better for us. As consumers, we have bought them, suffered our way through them and have never been more confused about what to eat.

In following Western dietary guidelines, we haven't just become victims of the same confusions and yo-yoing we see in the West, but we've also given up our own food wisdoms, handed down through the generations by the women in our homes. We started by avoiding fat in our diet, but only the naturally existing sources of fat. No ghee, no makhan, and surely no deep-fried bhajiya, not even when it's raining outside and the whole house is smelling of adrak chai. But it's okay to spread almond butter on bread, go for workshops that teach you how to cook Indian food in olive oil and chew on biscuits jiske har bite mein fibre hai. As long as it's making money for the food industry, it is backed by the doctor, dietitian, even the liftman. And from the educated to the illiterate, everyone looks down upon the local.

Your grandmother knows that if you are eating an egg, you should eat it the way the hen laid it, with the yellow and the white, both. If you are drinking milk, drink it the way the cow gave it, with its essential fats, probiotic bacteria and fat-soluble vitamins. If you are eating a fruit, eat one that's in season. But diet advice, at least the way we know it, won't have a word of this. Only egg whites, fat-free or low-fat milk, kiwis and the like rule the roost.

Nutrition colleges in India echo these confusions. Currently, the top two nutrition colleges in India are only for women. Not that marks are a sign of intelligence, but you also don't need to be a high-scorer to get admission to a nutrition course. Essentially, your talent pool is limited. And once you do make it to the course, you study things that have no cultural resonance and which are based on dividing food into calories and nutrients.

You can win a contest for the best protein meal by coming up with a recipe of rajma-paratha—it doesn't matter if no one has ever heard of it in your country. If you can, on paper, make it protein-rich, then you win. You are not expected to think of taste, much less assimilation of nutrients or excretion of waste. No thought spared for the time-tested rajma-chawal. No representation of what women at home know. No space for grandma's wisdom. No competition on traditional recipes. And incidentally, most competitions are sponsored by the food industry.

Eating right—according to the *Hatha Yoga Pradipika*—is an art, and the one who eats in a state of balance, called mitahar, is truly wise. This yoga or the oral wisdom that has stood the test of time finds no representation in nutrition or medical colleges. The syllabus revolves around what the West knows about food. You are systematically taught to look down upon what you learnt at home and are raised on a diet of science which changes itself all too often.

Doctors who study nutrition for a few weeks don't tire of giving us nutrient-based guidelines. So we come back home with advice to 'eat protein, avoid sugar, limit fat intake'—basically confused about what food we should actually eat and avoid. So we switch to oats for breakfast at the cost of poha, soup instead of dal-chawal and eat Marie biscuits with chai that has no sugar.

Take the average meal a dietitian prescribes in a weight-loss regime—soups, salads, steamed vegetables, whole grains over refined. Yet we do know that:

1. Soups are not a traditional part of our diet; they never needed to be. Vegetables lose nutrients with heat, while pulses retain it. Thus, native cultures have a liquid preparation of dals, and not of vegetables.

2. Vegetables naturally have what is known as anti-nutrients, molecules that can come in the way of nutrient assimilation, especially that of minerals. Cooking them, especially with herbs, spices and essential fat, read tadka, is a way of reducing the amount of anti-nutrients.
3. Excess consumption of fibre only washes away gut bacteria, putting us in a constant loop of constipation and loose motions. The rice we traditionally ate was hand-pounded white rice, not fibre-rich brown rice.

i could go on and on. But let me summarise simply. The big-picture view of our culture was not first propagated by some noble scientist. It came from an unbroken chain of commitment that passed food wisdom from generation to generation, like the guru-shishya parampara. These wisdoms came from our climate, the produce that grew here and our way of life. Just eating idli-chutney, dosa-sambar or dal-rice gives us a vegan, gluten-free, complete protein diet, but it doesn't sound as sexy as quinoa salad with cranberries, for example.

Traditional foods also promoted diet diversity. Depending on where you come from, you might eat paratha, poha or idli for breakfast. Now we all eat oats whether we are Malayali or Punjabi.

Nutrition experts across the world are now waking up to the fact that food science needs to be an interdisciplinary study that allows adequate learning from agriculture, economics and history, or else be willing to be written off as cuckoo science. The recently concluded FENS conference in Berlin, Europe's biggest nutrition conference, had a panel discussion that said food must be looked at as a system—farmer, trader, consumer, and not carb, protein, fat. That the only way to tackle the double burden of malnourishment is to put the focus on diversity of diets, encouraging populations to eat local, fresh, seasonal, and cook in a way that has cultural resonance. And that we have to put the traditional eating wisdoms, usually safeguarded by women in the past, at the centre of our understanding of food.

The unfashionable roti-sabzi, bhakri-sabzi, dal-rice, etc., is now considered a fool-proof way of getting good nourishment, while also being sensitive to local economies and carrying the tag of sustainability for the global ecology. The grandmother and her common sense is the repository of this interdisciplinary study, way ahead of its time and more than worthy of your time. It's the first open data source that we are exposed to, one that needs no wi-fi to download. Will we pay attention? That's the only question.

Fat loss, not weight loss

'You know, my neighbour, he is, like, stick-thin and he just went through a coronary bypass!' Heard that before, or know someone who's far from overweight and yet stuck with one or the other of those 'obesity-related diseases'? It's no surprise if you do. Though many of us jump on the weight-loss bandwagon to 'fix' a bad knee or back, blood pressure problems, diabetes and so on, these issues are not exclusive to overweight people. Those within the 'healthy body weight or BMI' range get them too. In fact, body weight is no indicator of fitness, health or wellness.

A more accurate marker of all three is your body composition. If your last 'successful' diet or exercise plan made you lighter on the scales and wallet but heavier on circulating body fat and poorer on lean body weight, you have only walked a step closer to heart disease and a host of other 'obesity-related' ailments. If your goal was to get healthier, and not to just lose weight because you have a wedding to attend, or because you are crossing forty, you need to get on to a sensible fat-loss plan.

The question is: how do we know that we are lowering our body fat levels and not just our body weight, when we drop kilos? i could write a book on that (in fact, i have) but here are some tell-tale signs that you have dropped fat, not just weight: Your nails will grow faster than ever. Your hair looks lustrous. You are able to lift and move things around effortlessly. You wake up hungry in the morning, and generally feel more in tune with hunger signals than before. And you no longer feel tired/bored about going to the gym or for a morning run.

Don't end up a TOFI!

i recently attended the International Sport Exercise & Nutrition Conference (ISENC) in Newcastle, where stalwarts of the industry (sports dietitians, exercise physiologists, trainers, sports medics, cardiologists) meet and share their learning with the rest of the world. The focus this year at the conference was the phenomenon of the medical and the weight-loss world reducing human beings to a number on the scale (body weight) and behaving as if there is no other physiological parameter that matters. This has not just been a major disservice to public health but also left many who have taken serious efforts to improve their health disappointed.

The consensus is that a focus on weight loss (or the lack of it) masks many, if not all, of the physiological (not to mention psychological) benefits that exercise and eating right bestows. The improved insulin sensitivity, endurance, strength, stamina, hunger cues, satiety signals, VO2 max, breathing rate, resting heart rate, better kidney and liver functioning, to name just a few. The term for people who don't lose weight on the scale but are otherwise leading a healthy, disciplined life is 'metabolically fit'. Their lifestyle ensures that they are not at risk of cardiac or any lifestyle-related disease.

One funky term for the metabolically fit is (i love this one) FOTI: Fat Outside, Thin Inside. And the term i love even more is TOFI: Thin Outside, Fat Inside, which acknowledges the fact that losing weight on the scale doesn't automatically reduce the risk of heart diseases, obesity, diabetes, etc. In fact, it can put you at a higher risk if the methods that led to the weight reduction were fundamentally incorrect—like starvation, over-exercise, surgeries or pills.

Haven't lost weight, but ...

... my energy levels are better
... my size is shrinking
... my skin is glowing

1. It's only when body fat is dropped that your body feels light (less lag on the body) and hence the increase in energy levels.
2. It's only when body fat is dropped that the volume shrinks, hence the drop in size. It may be accompanied by a gain in lean body weight and so no drop in weight.
3. It's only when body fat is dropped and lean body weight is higher that the insulin sensitivity picks up. This often leads to your skin (the largest organ of the body) looking healthier and fresher.

Sleep, caffeine and weight loss

The most underrated aspect of weight loss and staying in great shape is sleep. Caffeine is one of the biggest culprits in reducing sleep quality and therefore interferes with your weight loss. Here are some things you can do:
1. No coffee/chai after 3–4 p.m.
2. Energy drinks (Red Bull, Monster, etc.) are hidden sources of caffeine. Especially dangerous for teenagers. Will come in the way of optimum bone mineral density and hormonal health.
3. Painkillers, weight-loss pills, decaf coffees, green teas and chocolates (yeah, dark chocolates too) are the other unknown sources of caffeine and can stall your weight-loss efforts by disrupting your natural sleep pattern.

The right way to lose weight

The essence of losing weight the right way is to focus on developing good habits and not on losing weight.

Good Habits

- Eat local, seasonal and traditional foods.
- Eat from kitchen and not from packets.
- Eat with all senses and with gratitude and not fear.
- Stay active all day. Sit less, move more.
- Minimum 150 mins of exercise every week.
- Fix a bedtime and wakeup time.
- Regulate gadget use, especially before sleeping.
- Pursue your hobbies and spend time with family.

→

Good Health

- Energy levels are high
- Sleep quality is good
- Digestion is smooth
- No acidity or bloating
- No PMS or Period pain
- Good skin and hair
- You feel like exercising.
- No sugar cravings
- Blood sugars are regulated
- Lipid profile is good

→

Weight loss

- Sustainable and not yo-yo
- Irreversible
- Reduction in fat mass
- Gain in lean body mass and bone mineral density

~10-15% loss of body weight in a year

LEARNING – FOCUS ON DEVELOPING GOOD HABITS

Video - bit.ly/rightwaytoloseweight

Bad Habits

- Confused about what to eat and what to avoid
- Loss of confidence and body image issues
- Liable to fall prey to latest diet fads
- Sleep cycle goes for a toss as hormones are not regulated.
- Exercise becomes a punishment and there is never time for it.
- Relationship with self and loved ones always under stress

←

Bad Health

- Sugar cravings and erratic hunger
- Skin becomes dull and hair start falling.
- Irritability and mood swings
- Low energy levels and poor sleep quality.
- Poor digestion, acidity, constipation & bloating.
- Weak bones and poor joint health
- Loss of sexual drive
- Period cycle is erratic
- Frequent injuries

←

Weight loss

- Focus on losing weight at all cost
- Loss of muscle and bone mineral density
- Invariably weight comes back and sometimes more than you lost.
- Becomes more and more difficult to lose weight

RUJUTA SAYS...

If only our grandmom would have said good on waist instead of good on taste we would have never quit our dal-chawal-ghee. ;-)

Dark chocolate is healthy. Red wine is healthy. Green tea is healthy. For profits, not for people.

If you like a flying kiss over the real thing, then i can understand your need to use the air fryer!

Choosing foods based on calories is like deciding how to talk to people based on their salary.

Education is not about speaking in English and getting healthier is not about losing weight.

Eating in a certain way to 'lose weight' and in another way to 'maintain' is like dating one guy but marrying another. Waste of time, emotions and intelligence.

1C. FOOD MYTHS

The good bad foods

'Vashudhaiva Kutumbakam', all of the earth is my family, is the cultural heritage we belong to and the other learning that it gives us is, 'Anna he purna Brahma'—Food is all-encompassing or constitutes the whole universe. It wasn't until the 1970s that modern nutrition science took over and Indians began to view food in parts—protein, carb, good fat, bad fat, etc. The confusion hasn't ended, only compounded. Recently *Time* magazine had the big bad butter on its cover with the headline that maybe the scientists got it all wrong, and butter isn't bad after all. But anyways, here's looking at how we got our native foods all wrong.

1. Rice: Yeah, you have heard of Paleo and are all for 'ancient' grains for losing weight, but you are blind to the fact that rice is the most ancient grain that humans, more specifically us Asians, cultivated and rejoiced in as a divine grain. But then what about the 'carbs'? Well, it's also got amino acids (protein building blocks), vitamins, minerals and, hold your breath, fibre. But only brown, right? No, hand-pounded, single-polished, white-looking rice is not just easy on the palette but also on the stomach. And yes, it's great for 'high sugar', 'diabetes', etc. Remember, you eat rice along with sabzi, dal, dahi, etc., so the glycaemic index drops naturally; you don't need to buy a specific brand of rice for that.

2. Ghee: Oh God, saturated fat! Here we go again, the food that was celebrated as the purest and richest by a

culture that huge numbers throng to study, is on the strict 'no-no' list of the dietitian/doctor. Unless of course you practice in the high streets of NYC/London; then you call it clarified butter and recommend it for post-partum weight/depression, heart health and mobilising stubborn fat stores.

3. Sugar: That sweeteners are bad news is old news, but what about other sugar substitutes that are 'natural'? For starters, cane sugar is natural, comes from grass and until the 18th century was regarded as a priceless spice, especially for memsahibs who wanted to prevent sun damage and ageing skins. The secret here is glycolic acid (or Alpha Hydroxy Acid, as your skin products put it), which moisturises your skin. So eat that ghee-shakkar-roti and avoid those 'carb-free', 'gluten-free', 'fat-free' muffins/cereals/bread. Your so-called 'health food' can carry sugar in unhealthy amounts.

4. Full-fat milk: Soon, the mainstream media is going to sing the glories of dairy because that's how this game is usually played. Banish a food for a decade and then turn it into a miracle for another. You have seen it all with soya, fat, carbs, etc. Milk, with its naturally high CLA content, is great not just for bones, but also for keeping wrinkles at bay. And yes, vitamin D is fat-soluble, so if milk has no fat or is low fat, those vitamin D shots aren't going to help, baby.

5. Full-fat curd: The fat is essential to absorb the fat-soluble vitamins A, E, D, K, all of which play multiple roles in our body, but to our current interest, they leave us with a glowing skin. Each one of these vitamins, along

with the 'good bacteria' and vitamin B12, give you not just a tight skin but a taut stomach too. Old news, but worth repeating, is that lack of in-house bacteria is going to bloat you up, big time. So don't suck your stomach in for every picture, just eat a bowl of home-set curd daily and then just smile at the camera.

6. Mango: For a country that celebrated mango as the king of fruits, and was gifted by nature with over 1,000 varieties of the fruit, its current reputation as 'bad', 'high sugar', 'high calorie', 'fattening' is not just out of tune with what the shastras believed in, but also with diabetic associations across the world. The ancient texts believe it to be an anti-ageing, therapeutic food, and the ADA says it's good for a sustained blood sugar release. So now what's keeping you from enjoying it?

7. Sitaphal: From ridding you of constipation to giving you good amounts of easily digestible calcium and iron, this fruit is exactly what you should be looking out for if you are worried about how bloated or fat you have become. The perfect antidote to a hectic, stressed-out lifestyle.

8. Banana: Athletes with a lean frame depend on this fruit for their life, literally. It gives life or zest not just to fatiguing muscles but also to the brain. Reach out for this fruit when you get mad hungry between 4 and 6 p.m.: great to taste and easy on the stomach too.

9. Coconut: 'Shreephal', the fruit of the gods, has the reputation of an obstacle remover because it can make you mentally calm and physically all charged up. Technically, it has medium chain triglycerides, the fatty acids that

endurance athletes swear by. And no, there is no need for any cholesterol scare—virgin coconut oil in 2014 is what virgin olive oil was in early 2000: the answer to heart health, stubborn weight and everything in between.

10. Peanuts: Some call it the world's healthiest food. Loaded with vitamin B, vitamin E and micro minerals, this is what you should be reaching out for, for your 'choti bhook', especially if you are chota or an adolescent. The folic acid is important for everyone, but especially to our young ones. Peanuts are also a good source of the phytonutrient resveratrol—exactly the same nutrient that allows red wine to be the toast of heart health.

11. Wheat: At one point, wheat was considered to have more protein than rice, so rice-eaters switched to rotis. Soon, in its very refined form, wheat turned up everywhere from breads and muffins to cereals. Then they told us about the big bad gluten, and we began frantically shopping for gluten-free alternatives. Now research tells us that people who have avoided gluten in the last five years are fatter than people who have consumed gluten. So wait, before you get further confused: rice-eaters eat rice, roti-eaters eat roti, and avoid packaged whether or not it is gluten free.

12. Groundnut oil: It ruled the roost for the longest time and then it got too LS to continue using it in the kitchen. But thankfully it's making a grand entry back into our life as cold-pressed/single-pressed/virgin groundnut oil rich in oleic and linoleic acid as the perfect combination of omega 3, 6, 9, and thus the answer to our increasing cholesterol issues.

13. Fried stuff: There is no barish ka mazaa without eating fried food—bhajiya preferably. Look around and you will see a world full of vitamin D deficiencies. Dig deeper and you discover that they have stopped frying, even occasionally. Now at the cost of repeating myself, vitamin D is fat-soluble, so in the absence of dietary fat, even if you bake yourself in the sun or take all those shots, you will still be deficient. So eat fried, eat at home and don't refry.

14. Cashews: Again the cholesterol scare jumps into our face. Well, it's vegetarian and hence cholesterol free. Also, you need cholesterol, so stop being paranoid. As for cashews, they are being looked at as an alternative remedy to beating depression and can also help reduce BP. The next time your boss screams, chew on these cashews, it will keep your BP down and mood high.

15. Salt: There really is something called as hyponatremia, where your body can suffer things like cramps, headache, even near death, because of too little sodium. Just like there's too much of a good thing, there is also too little of a bad thing. Sodium is essential to keep the body's sodium–potassium pump in a healthy state, for your heart to beat and the legs to feel healthy. So don't avoid salt, avoid packaged foods.

16. Paneer: Old news, but paneer has protein, essential fat and vitamins too. So it's not fattening, nor will it increase your cholesterol, but not receiving adequate amounts of these nutrients from your diet will surely make you fat.

17. Pickle: Before you scream 'too much salt, too much oil', know that the salt and oil needs to be there so that

only the right kind of bacteria, the gut-friendly one, grows and that which is harmful dies. No need to buy all those probiotic milk/curd drinks after all; your grandmom's magic pickle is all you need, not just full of health, but love too.

18. Egg yolk: Everyone's favourite part in the egg, but the one that people have started avoiding because it is full of fat. Phospholipid (PL) is a special kind of fat, the fat that protects your heart and lowers your cholesterol—and scientists first discovered it in the yolk, the same egg yolk you avoid. PL has not just proved itself to be useful against inflammatory responses of the body that lead to high cholesterol, diabetes and ageing, but also in prevention of memory loss.

19. Chickoo: Heard of IBS, the inflammatory bowel syndrome? It wouldn't be wrong to say that almost everyone living an urban life is suffering from this to some extent. Chickoo can really come to the rescue and help us against this fast-spreading disorder. It contains polyphenolic compounds that help secrete certain gastro-intestinal enzymes that help improve metabolism. Basically, if you are trying to lose weight, surely eat the chickoo.

20. Sugarcane juice: There isn't a saint in Maharashtra that hasn't literally sung the glories of sugarcane. India's most trusted liver-cleanser in every situation, from a bad stomach to a jaundice attack, sugarcane, both juiced and chewed upon, is good for the entire gastrointestinal tract from mouth to anus. And yes, a sweet remedy against acne and pimples too.

Most common food myths

i) Ghee

The goodness of ghee

Ghee occupies the unenviable position as one of the most misunderstood foods in India today. At one time considered the food of Gods, it's now a 'fattening' ingredient and somehow responsible for the lifestyle diseases of this generation. But is that the truth? Since the 1970s and 1980s, when inspired by the marketing and propaganda of 'heart-healthy' vegetable oils an entire country let go of its 5,000-year-old food wisdom to eat ghee, has our heart health really improved? Are there fewer cases now of diabetes, high cholesterol, etc.? Or did we make a blunder when ghee was labelled harmful and pushed in the same category as trans-fats and hydrogenated fats?

Here is a summary of The Goodness of Ghee series from my Facebook posts:

Things we don't know or don't bother to know about ghee	**Most common myths about ghee and why you should banish them**
Ghee has antibacterial and antiviral properties. Other than helping you recover from sickness, it ensures that you don't fall sick.	*Ghee is fattening*. Ghee by nature is lipolytic, that which breaks down fat. And this is due to its unique short chain fatty acid structure.

Things we don't know or don't bother to know about ghee	**Most common myths about ghee and why you should banish them**
The antioxidants in ghee make it the miraculous anti-wrinkle and anti-ageing therapy you were searching for.	*Ghee is a saturated fat.* It's a saturated fat, yes, but with such a unique structure that it actually helps mobilise fats from stubborn fat area's of the body. Not a saturated fat like the trans-fats in your biscuits, cakes, pizza, etc.
Ghee is excellent for joint health, as it lubricates and oxygenates them.	*Ghee will increase cholesterol.* Ghee reduces cholesterol by increasing the contribution of lipids towards metabolism. Liver produces excess cholesterol under stress. Ghee helps you de-stress, sleep better and wake up fresher.
Ghee takes nutrients from your food and delivers them through fat-permeable membranes, like in the brain.	*Ghee is harmful for heart health.* Rich in antioxidants, conjugated linoleic acid (CLA) and fat-

Things we don't know or don't bother to know about ghee	**Most common myths about ghee and why you should banish them**
	soluble vitamins like A, E, D, ghee has just what you need for a healthy heart.
Ghee improves your satiety signal and ensures you eat the right amount of food.	*Okay, okay fine, ghee is good, but must not eat it too much.* Traditionally we add ghee in each meal. The quantity at which the taste of food is best is the right quantity. Only your tongue and stomach can tell you that.

P.S.: And yes, the best ghee is the one made at home from an Indian cow's milk. The next decent option is ghee from buffalo milk. The Jersey cow milk ghee has none of the benefits that you seek. So, that rules out tetra-packed milk. What you can do is support a goshala and help preserve the Indian cow.

For people outside India: Use the best possible option, but start making a demand for Indian cow milk/butter. Especially if you are in a country where 'customer is the king'.

The miracle food of India—ghee and its FAQs

Q: Why is ghee important for one's diet?

It's one of India's heritage recipes and a therapeutic one at that. The method in which ghee is made gives it a unique colour, consistency, flavour and aroma, along with multiple health benefits. So, from good looks to sharp brains, from overcoming constipation to spiritual evolution, ghee is celebrated in India for every reason—gross to subtle, small and big.

Q: What are the health benefits of having ghee?

Great skin, lubricated joints, stronger immune function, better memory, heart health, fertility, anti-carcinogenic and everything in between. Super crucial these days for assimilation of vitamin D, because vitamin D deficiency is the rich man's new disease.

Q: How much ghee should one have in a day?

As much as one wants, as much as is required to bring out the best taste, flavour, aroma and texture of food without making it greasy. The right quantity also depends on what you are eating, e.g. dal baati or bajra roti will need more ghee compared to dal-rice or khichdi.

Q: The market is abuzz with many types of ghee. What type of ghee should one have?

The one that is made at home following all the protocols—being distilled or purified from milk to malai, from malai to butter, and then churned and heated—is the best one. The important thing to remember here is that the milk should come from the Indian breed of cows, often called desi cow and the one that walks around and grazes on nutritious grass. Not the Jersey cow that you saw in the DDLJ movie, which is fed corn and hormones.

Q: There is also an alternative debate that ghee has disadvantages for people who are overweight, and also leads to cardiovascular diseases. How would you respond to that?

The debate exists because people confuse ghee with any other saturated fat. Just like they have now learnt that all fat is not bad, they will also learn that all saturated fat is not the same. While it makes sense to avoid saturated fat that comes in 'fibre-rich' biscuits and 'iron-enriched' cereals, it is important to understand that the saturated fat in ghee is different from the one that is found in packaged and processed food products. Ghee has a very unique carbon atom structure, much smaller than the usual, commonly found and rightfully feared saturated fat. This unique carbon atom chain is what gives ghee all its therapeutic, almost magical, properties. The 'debate' is a consequence of half information, one that overlooks the basics of chemistry.

Q: How should one include ghee in everyday diet?

Ghee is versatile in nature; it can lend itself beautifully to deep frying, tadka or can be added to flavour dals, rotis, parathas, etc. You could even apply it to your toes or head as a relaxant and it works better than a sleeping pill. Its smoking point is high, so you can have it cold, warm or hot, depending on individual preference and the type of cuisine involved.

ii) Coconut

Why you must have coconut

So fortunate that my window looks out to the kalpavruksha (wish-fulfilling tree), coconut. And so heartbroken that it has been downgraded to a palm/grass by the Goa government.

1. Every part of the coconut tree helps humanity.
2. It takes salinity from the ground water and turns it to nectar like coconut water.
3. Addition of coconut to food helps reduce the glycaemic index of the meal.
4. The medium chain triglycerides in the coconut help improve heart health and reduce cholesterol levels.
5. Tender coconut water is nature's own sports drink with the electrolyte balance that prevents blood pressure and works like a detox in the body.

Nariyal pani

You want to truly chill in the heat? Forget the fizzy drinks that dehydrate you, the fruit juices drained of fibre and vital nutrients, and instead grab the world's most natural and ultimate cold drink. No, i am not launching a new product, i am talking about the humble nariyal pani. No added flavours, additives, sugars, colours, just 100 per cent natural sugar and an impressive electrolyte ratio.

These electrolytes in the nariyal pani not only help you restore your sodium–potassium balance and hydration levels, but also leave your skin looking fresh and acne-free in the summer heat. The wonders of this drink never get advertised as the best thing for your child or for your waist. Maybe because when something is truly natural (and cheap), we stop caring about it and focus on artificial things that we can market as 'natural' and make more money in the bargain? The drink falls 'short' on another front too—it's not well packaged. It comes in a hard shell of a coconut and not in some fancy can with a label that says low-cal/natural/packed with potassium power. And then there is the malai, 'fattening' and 'saturated', as per your health practitioner. Tsk tsk. This saturated fat found in nariyal is so unique in its structure that it helps (hold your heart) protect your heart from cardiovascular diseases, improves your stamina, nourishes your skin and hair and aids in burning fat. Not to mention, both the pani and the malai are just great to taste.

The making and un-making of the coconut oil controversy

The West in general and the US in particular will stumble upon a 'novel' food and then it's everywhere, in their cuppa as bullet proof coffee, in their blueberry pastry as a vegan dessert, or even as a shot to drink first thing in the morning to kick-start metabolism. Yeah, that's the pedestal that coconut oil was on until last week and this is after being non-existent in their food chain until ten years ago.

Not just coconut oil, staple foods from developing economies have often caught the fancy of the developed world because of their nutrients—medium chain triglycerides in the case of coconut, protein for quinoa, antioxidants for turmeric. Some paperwork, a few lab studies, the right pitches to the mainstream media, and this novel food is then everywhere, dominating the health food stores, social media feeds and kitchen cabinets. It is basically the answer to every problem you have had, until of course it is not. The recent coconut oil controversy aside, this cycle will continue for as long as we look at food from the nutrient point of view, and only that.

It's easier said than done of course. Studying and knowing food from only the nutrient point of view is good for business and the food industry is well entrenched in our education system. A nutrition graduate or postgraduate invests three to five years in the study of food as nothing but its nutrients and calories. A doctor studies the same thing but over a single semester, and everyone giving you food advice is now on the same page. What is left out of the syllabus is crop cycle, climate, regional cuisines. So are agriculture, economy, ecology. This way you have zero exposure and understanding of the real environment you will be working in. You step out of college, you rehash the information you learnt there, advice people accordingly, and the mainstream media backs you too.

So, no one blinked an eyelid when in the 1970s, you were asked to go off coconut because of cholesterol and ghee because of saturated fat and to use refined vegetable oils instead. Forty years later, refined vegetable oils are toxic and you should go back to coconut and ghee, and then don't, it's poison. Well, i will tell you what is poison: the mentality to reduce food to nutrients and then adopting or rejecting it. Activist and author Michael Pollan calls it nutritionism; it's the systemic vilification of food so that food companies may profit while public health suffers.

In an increasingly global world, just like we unite against racism, sexism and ageism, we should do the same against nutritionism. We should eat foods because they are native to our land, are culturally compliant and are in season. And eat them in the multiple ways we have learnt to. In the case of coconut, it would mean—when it's tender, you drink its water; when it's ripe, you use it as garnish or as stuffing in delicacies; use dry coconut in laddoos and barfis; and the oil for cooking if you are in Kerala or are a Malayali. (By the way, Kerala, which is known for its consumption of coconut, has a healthy ageing population—it has the most number of people in their nineties as compared to the rest of India.)

As for saturated fat, the science is out there. There is no evidence to conclusively link saturated fat to heart disease but there is plenty to link consumption of ultra-processed and packaged food to obesity and a host of other diseases including heart diseases. Ever read a headline that said 'Chocolate, chips, colas are pure poison'? i haven't yet.

But for me, just like the coconut, life has come a full circle. When i started working twenty years ago, if the West carried an article saying one of our native foods is poison, our media would copy it and my clients would question why i was insistent on feeding them poison. Today, everyone is questioning the headline—to me, that's the best news of the decade.

iii) Sugar

Why sugar is not your enemy

The fifty-year-old actress who once stole your heart is now running after an eight-year-old boy with a bowl of chocolate-coated cereal. She's playing a mother to a fussy boy for whom the cereal seems to be the only source of nourishment. They don't explicitly show it, but in your head, you have already imagined that the bowl has low-fat milk. Thankfully, the boy has the meal, he loves it in fact, and the two celebrate by playing a video game.

Another fifty-year-old actor overcomes mountains, traffic and death itself to pick a bottle of what the EU calls SSB or sugar-sweetened beverage. That essentially expands the list beyond the colas to include packaged fruit juices, probiotic yoghurt drinks, energy and sports drinks.

Kids from Class IX hang out at cafés sipping monstrously big glasses of cold coffee or choco shakes after tuition classes. When they study, they quickly make themselves some noodles or pasta in two minutes. They watch TV programmes interspersed with ads that ask them to mix powders in milk to grow taller, run faster or simply look cooler.

All of the above have tons of sugar, but i hope you are beginning to realise that sugar is hardly the problem. The product, positioning and pricing is. That our kids are moving less on bikes and sitting more is. That we reduce fifty-year-old women to aunties and fifty-year-old men to dudes is. That we don't have a policy on how junk food should be advertised is. That we don't tax food companies or hold them accountable for the garbage that they create with their packets, tetra-packs and bottles is. Pick on the big guys and leave the ragpickers of Deonar alone, man. But that's not how this works.

So instead of looking at the picture in totality we reduce our problem to sugar. Sugar is the enemy. Sugar is killing us. Sugar is making us fat. Sugar is giving us diabetes and the likes. Isn't there a word for it—deflection? Or hey! Don't change the subject if you are just a middle class, angrezi-speaking Indian like me. We like intelligence sold to us in easy-to-understand terms. We are sure that governments cannot be held accountable, food companies are above the law—probably even making the law—and we are too short on time for any kind of activism. If we look at the total problem, we don't know what to do. But if we have something fairly simple to make a lifestyle choice with, we will adopt it.

So, no more sugar for me in the chai but i will have a Marie biscuit to go with it. Marie or digestive is a healthy choice because it's not as sweet as a regular biscuit. There you go, the sweetness is the problem. So no more sugary fruits like mango, sitaphal, jackfruit, chickoo, etc. Doesn't matter if they are local, doesn't matter if they contain natural fruit sugar, fructose. The American Diabetic Association can recommend mango to diabetics but in the land of its origin, it is banned by doctors and dietitians. We aren't outraged about it on social media. We are quite cool about the banistan as long as it is about all local fruit and produce in general.

The sugar substitute market is expected to reach $16.53 billion in 2020. This growth is driven by the health-conscious modern consumer in the West, and the demands of the health and personal care industry of developing countries like India and China.

In the meanwhile, Hillary Clinton and Bernie Sanders fought over soda tax in their presidential campaigns and the UK levied soda tax from April 2018. What we must consider before buying into the West's fear of sugar is that nutrition science as we knew it—where everything can be split into categories such as carb, protein, fat or calories—is changing. Food scientists the world over are acknowledging the fact that there is more to food than these categories.

Sugar to India is as ancient as yoga and Ayurveda itself. It is one of the panch amrits, or nectars of life. What has changed is the way India consumes its sugar. Being a native plant, we have had the sophistication to use the plant in diverse, versatile ways depending on the season and region. From Diwali to Sankranti, there are festivals that celebrate the power of sugarcane because that is also harvest time. Apart from taste, sugarcane has fibre, mineral and vitamins. It's also a folk remedy for jaundice. Sugarcane juice boiled with pulses is an inexpensive but complete meal for the tribals of western Maharashtra.

Jaggery and ghee combinations along with bajra and other millet rotis are known to provide the body with warmth and the joints with mobility in the harsh north Indian winter. In Bengal, sweet, delicate sandesh is known to lift the spirits of even cynical leftists. The mishri-saunf combo works as a digestive aid in summer. And the crystalline sugar is in everything, from prasad to a sharbat.

None of the traditional ways in which we use sugar is depicted in ads or marketing campaigns. Why must we give up on the traditional uses of sugar and use packaged products that use sugar substitutes?

India now consumes three times more sugar than it used to just in the 1970s, and that's not because it's eating more mithai or adds more sugar in chai. But because it's drinking more colas, packaged juices and eating sugared cereals. It is distributing brownies, cupcakes and frozen yoghurts instead of dry fruits, laddoos and mithai during Diwali. It is patronising food products of big companies and not the small women-run enterprises that make mithai. It is funding the third house or the private jet that the food company's CEO is buying and not the dance class the daughter of a small entrepreneur who makes puran poli wants to attend. Sugar is not the problem, giving up on food traditions without a thought is.

Sweet nothings

It's time to bust the myth that sweeteners help you consume less calories and lose weight. The reality is: your total calorie consumption goes up the moment you choose a sugar substitute over sugar.

Try this experiment. Take a good look at what fat people put into their chai/coffee, and what thin people add to theirs. Typically, it's not the thin people but the fat uncles and aunties who habitually add sweeteners. Ever wondered why they remain fat? The answer is that the chemicals in sweeteners cause changes in the pH balance (acidity levels) of the body, and that makes them crave more food. Also, you may fool the brain with 'pretend sugar', but when you don't generate the energy it associates with the consumption of 'real' sugar, the brain rebels and asks you to eat more. So does your satiety centre, quite upset at being cheated. That's why sweetener-addicts end up eating cookies loaded with trans-fat with their tea.

It's the same with diet colas. Gullible teenagers don't realise what these 'zero-calorie' drinks do to their systems. They also think 'saving' sugar calories makes it okay to splurge on the high-calorie pizza or burger consumed with the cola. Get real. Losing fat involves way more than the math of calories. It involves the chemistry of tiny molecules in your body; the history of your past meals and workouts; the geography of your location; the physics of the actual mass of food you consume at one time. So put that spoon of sugar into your tea or coffee; even if calories haunt you, it's only twenty calories; you probably burnt that much by just reading this piece. One gulab jamun or peda won't kill you either. What will harm you is that nutrient-bereft pizza, burger, cookie or cake that you ate unthinkingly. And that sweetener you virtuously put into your tea.

iv) Mango

Go man, mango!

Look up and you will see the signs all around you. Flowers blooming on the trees, birds singing their song and the king of fruits declaring that he will arrive in all grandeur shortly. So, here's a factsheet on mango that you must be aware of before the season begins, so that you relish the fruit in its full glory and be well-equipped to fight the propaganda of doctors, dietitians and trainers that mango is fattening, high on sugar, etc.

• Mango for diabetes? YES! Diabetics are asked to eat foods that are low on the glycaemic index. The glycaemic index is a measure of how quickly your blood sugar rises in response to the food you have consumed. Now mango has a low GI, just like apple and berries. So why is apple 'allowed' and mango not? i am guessing mango is tastier. And while the American Diabetic Association recommends mango for diabetics, our doctors—who love flaunting their foreign degrees—ensure that you stay away from the fruit a small farmer sells and instead go for biscuits that huge corporations sell. Tch tch.
• Mango for high cholesterol? Yes. The pectin, that soluble fibre, is so great for lowering cholesterol levels and so much yummier than the oats you eat. i mean why tolerate the poor taste of oats for fibre when a yummier mango is at hand?
• Mango for blood pressure? Yes! They are an amazing source of polyphenols, the same reason why you drink copious amounts of green tea, however bland or yucky it tastes. So these polyphenols protect the heart against damage, and you want that if you have blood pressure issues.

Proudly be an aam admi

Mango! Yay! Is what you should be saying, but if you are fearful of all local fruits, be it the sitaphal, chickoo, banana, grapes or jackfruit, you most likely have the following concerns:

1. My doctor asked me to avoid mango.

If he/she also asked you to avoid the fruits above and instead eat apples, berries, kiwis, oranges and melons, simply disregard the advice. It stems not from facts but lack of value and knowledge (bordering on fear) of anything local.

2. But it's too sweet!

Sweetness is the virtue of a fruit, don't turn it into a villain.

3. But i have diabetes.

Mango is low (or moderate) and not high on the glycaemic index. It's safe. Fruits that are low to moderate on the glycaemic index are recommended for pre-diabetic, diabetic, insulin-insensitive cases. What about cholesterol? Rich in fibre, pectin (a natural bio-polymer), vitamin C and vitamin B, they together have a beneficial effect on your lipid profile. In simple words, it will reduce your cholesterol levels. Psst ... the same dietitian who tells you not to eat mango is likely to push for oats for its 'fibre-rich' properties. While oats are sold by large food companies, mangoes are sold by small farmers. i rest my case.

4. i am a heart patient.

Rich in antioxidants like beta carotene, vitamin B6 and minerals like zinc, copper, manganese, mango actually has the power to reduce the effects of free radicals (damaging to the heart and other organs) in your body. That's also the reason it is steadily gaining popularity as an anti-carcinogen.

Celebrate the mango, and relish it not just for its nutritional properties but for its taste, sweetness and incomparable richness.

5. What about artificial ripening/carbide in mangoes?

Food adulteration is a big issue and while we should ask for greater accountability in how our food is produced, procured and stored, we should also take active steps to get more involved in our food environment.

Here are some easy steps you can adopt:

• Buy mango only once the season starts (e.g. post Akshaya Tritiya in the south and west).

• Buy the local mango of your region (we have over a thousand different varieties in the country). More local, less likely it is to be adulterated.

• Buy directly from a farm (wherever possible) or patronise the trusted aam wala who will have all the checks in place on your behalf.

You can also form a small group of like-minded people and place your order together, which will give the farmer an incentive to come and deliver directly to you.

Last but not the least, do know that amongst the most adulterated fruit in the market in terms of chemicals used is the apple.

Yeh koi aam baat nahi—the mango speaks out

The farmer battles unpredictable weather, water shortage and declining soil health to grow the mango. All he hopes for is a good harvest and a decent price for the produce. The money generated from it goes towards the education, health and food for his family. There is no money to sponsor medical or nutrition conferences, to rope in actors, chefs and other influencers to be their brand ambassadors or spokesperson. There is no association of farmers, and if they do have one, they are not influential or backed by governments and industries. And so, for years we have believed that not just the mango but almost all our local fruits, like sitaphal, banana, jackfruit, chickoo, grapes, etc., are bad for us.

But nutrition scientists now say that patronising local food is important for public health, local economy and global ecology. Want to lose weight and get rid of your diabetes? Get off your seats, switch off your phones, close your eyes and bite into the mango. Aam karta hai sab gile shikve maaf.

Mango 101

Native fruit, cultivated for over 6000 years
Over 1500 varieties known
India largest producer,
US, Netherlands, UK, France Germany biggest importers

Heart & cholesterol

Rich in fibre and Vitamin C, helps in digestion and regulates blood lipid levels. Good for cholesterol.

Abundance of vitamins, minerals and enzymes that have a cardio protective effect, reduce risk of heart disease

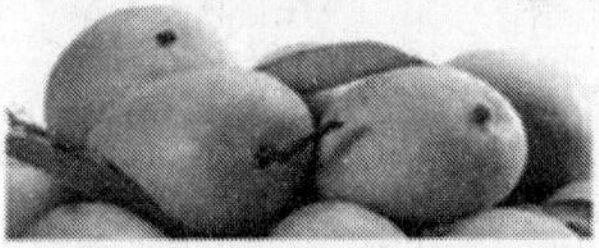

Diabetes & cancer

Mangiferin, a bioactive compound found in Mangoes, has multiple therapeutic benefits and is used in treatment of infections, diabetes, cancer, heart disease.

World wide, Diabetic associations recommend eating fresh, seasonal fruits including Mangoes.

Known in Ayurved, Chinese medicine, East Asia and even Cuba for its anti-bacterial, anti-viral, anti-diabetes and anti-cancer properties

And more

- Zeaxanthin and carotene, protect the eyes and skin from free radical damage and ageing
- Rich in Vit B, helps in production of red blood cells, good for the brain and improves fat burning
- Dense in phenolic compounds, helps prevent liver damage, inflammation and chronic conditions including obesity

Glycaemic index 51 or lower
Above 55 is considered high.

Glycaemic load of 12.8
Above 20 is considered high

Protects eyes
Rich in fibre
Vitamin C
Helps in digestion
Regulates blood lipid levels
Good for cholesterol
Anti-viral
Anti-bacterial
Prevent liver damage
Vitamin B
Fat burning
Anti-diabetes
Anti-cancer properties
Therapeutic benefits
Anti-ageing
Protects skin

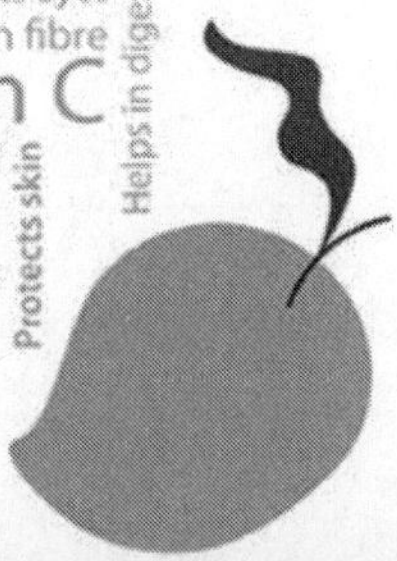

Rujuta Diwekar

v) Rice

Rice is nice

Rice is a perfect example of the weight-loss industry (with the aid of 'research and marketing') brainwashing entire cultures into believing the food that they have always eaten is somehow harming them. World over, nutrition bodies have finally recognised this phenomenon as 'nutrient transition', where ancient communities are becoming increasingly prone to diabetes, obesity, heart and other lifestyle diseases after switching from their local, seasonal foods to something exotic, non-native.

Here is a summary of the Rice is Nice series.

Things we don't know or don't bother to know about rice	**Most common myths about rice and why you should banish them**
It promotes growth of probiotic bacteria, eases bowel movement and rids you of bloating.	*Rice has starch.* a) Cooked rice has less than 10 per cent starch and b) Starch is a source of energy as it's converted to glucose in the body, so we need it.
It prevents premature wrinkles.	*Rice is high GI and bad for diabetics.* Rice, as it is traditionally eaten with dal/sabzi/meat/dahi, etc., reduces the GI of the meal and is great for diabetics.

Things we don't know or don't bother to know about rice	**Most common myths about rice and why you should banish them**
It has essential amino acids like methionine, which when consumed with dal, for example, completes the amino acid profile of the meal. (They are limiting factors of each other.)	*Rice is carbs, so avoid, especially at night.* a) No food is just carbs or proteins or fats b) Rice has crucial amino acids, vitamins and many phytonutrients c) Carbs are essential for our body and have a calming effect, therefore great as a dinner option.
Has inositol, which has fat-burning, anti-anxiety, and irritability reducing properties.	*Brown is better than white.* a) Traditionally we have always eaten hand-pounded or single-polished rice, which is whitish, not brown b) This kind of rice lets the body assimilate all the nutrients from it, e.g. vitamin B6.
It allows for better assimilation of vitamin D and calcium.	*Okay, okay fine, rice is nice, but must not eat it too much.* Too much of hawa is also bad, so completely let go of your fear of rice, eat it and trust your tongue and stomach to guide you.

Myths about rice stem from basically two reasons: a) Ignorance about the wisdom surrounding food passed down over generations. Not just ignorance, but disdain almost. b) Knowing little about the science behind food. No one claims to be an expert in fields like CA, engineering, design, medicine, etc., etc., but for some reason everyone is one when it comes to nutrition. So things like carbs are bad, or rice has starch or it's fattening, are nothing but fantasies of a brain starved of, ironically, carbs and fats.

Eat your rice the way you like it, eat it as often in the day as you want and eat it in quantities which will leave you feeling light and energetic, and enjoy the wonders it will bring to your body.

P.S.: This post was in part motivated by misleading ad campaigns that claim that their rice is fibre-rich or cholesterol-free or has a low glycaemic index, which gives the general public an impression that the regular rice they have traditionally been eating doesn't have all these benefits.

How the (food) fear spreads

Recently a newspaper headline screamed: 'South India worst hit by diabetes; rice to be blamed?' Now i would have learnt in a journalism school that it's exactly this kind of 'statement' that makes a headline. (a) It is clear you are encouraged to not be clever (b) It is relevant to a rice-eating nation, something which Google results can grab and (c) It stirs the reader emotionally. 'Oh no! i should really not eat that thairsadham after all.' Chalo toh full marks to the report. Well done!

The truth is that most of us read 'news' like this—headline to headline. We don't bother reading the actual report, we are in a rush and we just want to quickly glance through what's happening in the world. It makes us feel smart, intelligent and 'with it'. So the smart, intelligent and cool people that we are, we quickly tell ourselves and everyone around us that rice is bad, fattening and now 'research' has 'proved' that it's the 'leading cause' of 'diabetes'.

And everyone is only too eager to believe all this. Fear sells like hot cakes, common sense is tough to sell. So if you were to read the report in detail, you'd see that the prevalence of diabetes in Kerala (8.83 per cent) and Andhra Pradesh (7.24 per cent) is lower than Tamil Nadu (11.76 per cent). Himachal (6.06 per cent), Uttarakhand (5.91 per cent) and Bihar (4.88 per cent) are much lower than the national average (7.1 per cent). But here is the thing—these states are predominantly rice-eating states. And what about Maharashtra? Poha, ghavan, pej, dahi bhat, waran bhat, masala bhat, modak—we eat rice in every form and in every course of our meal. So we must be high on this list, right? Nope, Maharashtra is 3.56 per cent, second lowest in the country.

So why didn't the headline read, 'Eating rice is great for diabetes?' Or that 'There is no link between rice and diabetes (even within this study design)?' Because this doesn't make for juicy news and you need something to grab eyeballs. And as a reader what you should ask yourself is, why do these kind of reports appear on the day or the week when some 'diabetes-free' or 'healthy' rice is being launched?

vi) Nuts

Nuts to heart-healthy oils!

The oil jar in your kitchen could well decide the number of stretch marks on your thighs and if you'll sport love handles on your waist. A wider girth means a greater risk of heart disease (old news, i know), and so we duly switched to heart-healthy oils and virgin olive oils. But even then, our girth keeps increasing, and so does our vulnerability to lifestyle diseases (old news, yes, but i'm not sure you noticed). So, which oil should you use?

Try filtered groundnut oil (or mustard, til or coconut depending on where you live). Look for the words 'filtered' or 'cold-pressed' or 'virgin' on the label. Filtered oil is extracted from the seed at a much lower temperature than refined oil. At low temperatures, the fatty acid bonds in the groundnut don't get destroyed, keeping its heart-protecting abilities intact, along with vitamins and minerals. This, however, makes oil extraction a little expensive as you don't get too much oil out of each seed while maintaining the quality. A cheaper way to make oil is to use high temperature, technology and solvents to extract a near-100 per cent yield out of the seeds. But this destroys the delicate fatty acid bonds and weakens naturally existing vitamins and minerals.

Though these oils are cheaper, they are sold at a higher price thanks to advertising. Filtered oils are almost never advertised and are more likely to be stocked at your grocer's rather than the mall. Filtered groundnut oil doesn't just have anti-viral properties, but is great for fat loss too. Groundnuts, with their high niacin (of the vitamin B family) content, help stabilise blood sugars and, thus, aid in fat loss. Eating groundnuts/peanuts is good for diabetics (i know you were advised against it) because its nutrient-rich properties also help prevent cardio-vascular complications. So, for a healthy heart, a strong immune system and fat loss, bring back good old groundnut oil. It was once a staple of your grandmom's kitchen, and that explains her glowing skin.

Cashew, coconut, copper

Cashews and coconut—both start with the letter 'c' but really that is no reason why it should give you the cholesterol scare. As for what 'they' say about cashews and coconuts, i think they are not exactly good at another 'c': chemistry.

So, isn't coconut 'full' of saturated fat? Yup, it is a rich source of saturated fat, but dig a little deeper, actually just scratch and apply some basic chemistry you learnt in school, and you will realise it's dominantly a medium chain triglyceride. MCTS, as they are known in the world of endurance sports like marathons and Tour de France, are a unique type of fat, easy on the stomach and quick to burn for more stamina and better recovery.

In the world of biochemistry, they are recognised as the special fat that helps improve the HDL or the 'good' cholesterol. Now you do know this but just to brush up, a high HDL to total cholesterol ratio is known to reduce risk of heart disease. So come on, garnish that sabzi with coconut and eat your idlis with your coconut chutney.

Continuing my love affair with cashews, it's rich in another 'c'—copper. Copper is an antioxidant that works at eliminating the free radicals from your body. Free radicals put you at a risk of developing hypercholesterolemia, heart disease and the like. Copper is also an integral part of an enzyme called lysyl oxidase, which allows for cross-linking of collagen and elastin and keeps your bones, joints and most importantly the blood vessels flexible and healthy.

And before you ask me to state my 'research', will you please dig up yours which allowed you to link coconut and cashews to cholesterol so 'c for conclusively'?

Love for cashew curry

Love, it can sweep you off your feet, fill the room with its fragrance and leave a good taste in your mouth for years to come. But when it comes, you should be ready to receive, with an open mind, open heart and a hungry stomach. Coz sometimes love comes in the form of kaju usal (tender cashew curry). And then you must remind yourself how lucky you truly are to have crossed paths. Most of the world won't even know what it means, looks like or tastes like. But it will fill you, fulfil you and leave you feeling full too. The latest diet recommendations for the world in the EAT-Lancet report says that we must eat more regional to show some love to ourselves and to our planet. And yet in our real lives diversity is compromised for homogeneity. The future beckons us to set ourselves free from the clutches of carb, protein, fat and embrace local, seasonal, traditional. Will we, is the only question.

CASHEW FRUIT

Five times richer in vitamin C than orange but still not taught as a source of vitamin C in our schools. Kaju deserves better. Let's call it the 'cashew apple' so that it sounds cool enough to possess all the antioxidant properties ;-).

The polyphenols in the kaju fruit give it a unique taste, kill bacteria that cause tooth decay and prevent mouth ulcers. If you have a child, make sure she eats at least one in the season.

Boiled groundnuts, the super legume, and why you must have them

1. Diabetics: Prevents leg pains and night cramps thanks to its mineral- and vitamin B-rich profile. Also helps regulate blood sugar.
2. Heart disease: The essential fatty acids and resveratrol (for which wine claims to be good for the heart) amongst many other antioxidants make it good for the heart and prevent free radical damage.
3. PCOD: The biotin, B1 and B6 help cut down bloating, PMS and prevent acne and hair loss.
4. Teenage: Protein-rich and full of micronutrients, it makes for a quick, inexpensive snack and keeps mood swings away.
5. Pregnancy: Expecting moms who eat peanuts regularly have better gut bacteria diversity that helps babies fight infections, allergies and intolerances better.

vii) Pickles/Papads

In the deepest pickle

We are happy to fuss over our organic/natural/vegan ways but look down on the poor little pickle. Pickles, after all, can't possibly have any health benefits with all the oils and salt they have. And if your grandmother fussed over it, made a loud noise about not touching that ceramic bottle with wet hands, tied up the neck with a malmal cloth and stored it in a special corner of the kitchen, it's a nuisance, not a fat-burning agent. And that it tastes good and is an accessible home-grown wisdom must surely make it fattening.

Cut to this morning. You have strained on the pot and your stomach doesn't feel as light as it should. A big reason for your digestive troubles is that stress and a fast-paced lifestyle could have destroyed the bacteria in your GI tract. This live bacteria is often called the 'good bacteria' and its health benefits range from great skin, smooth stools, regular BP and lowered blood sugars.

Your grandmom knows that vegetables and fruits can be cultured or treated using a mixture of sugar, oil, salt, mustard, cumin, etc. to prepare the right strain and strength of the probiotic bacteria. She knows that it must be stored in the right environment to prevent humidity leading to the oxidation and destruction of this bacterial culture. She also knows that if it is consumed in small doses, as part of a wholesome meal, it will reach the gut alive without being destroyed by the stomach acids.

The only thing she doesn't know is that if she wants you to eat it, she should brand it as fat-burning, give it an exotic name and charge you millions for it. By the way, the process she is using is called lacto fermentation by 'research'.

Pickles—fears and facts

Fear—pickle is full of salt and oil.
Fact—without the oil and salt, the gut-friendly bacteria won't grow and you won't have all the benefits of pickle.
Fear—the salt will cause BP.
Fact—it's not salt that causes BP, it's habits like lack of exercise, poor sleep hygiene and packaged, processed foods that cause it. Use unprocessed jada or kala or sendha namak as per your food heritage.
Fear—oil is not good for heart health.
Fact—consumption of fat or oil doesn't cause heart problems, it's habits (refer to the fact related to BP above). Use kacche ghani ka groundnut, mustard, til or gingley oil according to your food heritage.
Fear—but pickle is unhealthy.
Fact—pickle is a storehouse of minerals, vitamins and friendly bacteria. One-two teaspoons of pickle every day can help reduce bloating, anaemia, vitamin D- and B12-deficiencies and is even helpful for IBS.
Conditions apply: ghar pe banao, pyaar se khao, ghabrau nako.

Papads

As the weight loss–food–pharma industries boomed, all native inventions, practices and foods were rubbished for being fattening or plain boring. Well, there's nothing boring or fattening about the many varieties of papad though, and here's why they should still occupy a place of pride in your kitchen.

1. Climate resilient: Uses the heat of summer to make food items that are sun-matured so that they can last and come to your rescue in the wet monsoons and cold winters.
2. Zero wastage: Uses everything from sabudana to dals, millets to potatoes, prepped in a way that retains nutrients and stays ready to cook as per demand. That way, on a rainy day, when your grandma didn't feel like toiling in the kitchen, these came to her rescue, completed her nutrient needs, satiated her. She didn't open her phone and call for food that came in packaging of plastic, cardboard and tissues. She went about her life without creating garbage (maybe that's why she looks better than you).
3. Gender neutral: If grandma employed her grandsons in making papads, she employed her husband, your grandpa, in frying them. She owned the good life, she didn't tear up when she saw her husband in the kitchen, she walked the talk of equality—i make dal chawal, you fry papads and clean up later.
4. The good life: Nothing feels better than dal-chawal or khichdi with a crackling, deep-fried papad crushed with your teeth. And you deserve the good life, the good taste and the good time. And you deserve it now, not after you have lost two sizes. Now. Because a narrow waist belongs to those who embrace their heritage with broad-mindedness.

viii) Dairy

Why it breaks my heart when i read about milk and cruelty to cows—and how food trends miss the bigger picture.

• Food is the foundation of fitness, and yet the narrative on food and fitness is totally disconnected from farming.

• Small farms, like the ones that most Indian farmers own, are an ecosystem by themselves. Farm animals like cows, goats, sheep, along with the earthworms, birds and bees and even the farming family itself live together as a wholesome unit. One nurturing and caring for the other.

• The cow, for example, is raised and treated like family by farmers, pretty much like how a pet gets treated at home. The calf always drinks first, and most farmers will only milk from one or two udders. To sustain their small farms, Indian farmers don't just have to use cow dung and urine but also sell milk.

• Milk, ghee, curd were and are part of the panch amrit across all regions in India. From the pind to the brahmanda or individual health to local economy to global ecology, they look after every aspect of wellbeing.

• Let's not turn into a junta who sees cruelty in milking cows but chomps down quinoa for protein, unaware of quinoa wars and rampant destruction of forests in the Amazon. Denying a farmer her/his due income is cruelty too; so is following a trend without checking its relevance to the region you live in.

To keep farming a viable option for our rural population, and to have access to good food for the urban population, we must connect to farms and farm animals.

“

RUJUTA SAYS...

A good diet is like true love, it sets you free.

If you would like a job with zero salary, then i can understand your need to eat zero calorie.

Crash diets are like fake jewellery, bure time mein aap ke kaam nahi aata! ;-)

The rage of today is garbage of tomorrow, especially true of diets and crushes.

Real food and true love come without labels and remorse.

If you are unable to stick to a diet in spite of your best intentions, it’s the diet’s fault not yours. A healthy diet must account for cultural, regional and personal preferences.

”

1D. DIET TRENDS

Diet according to the Bhagwad Gita

Would have meals that lead to:

• Ayuh, satva, bala, arogya—long life, vitality, strength, health.

• Karmesu kaushalama—excellence in your chosen path/work.

• Yukta aharasya, chetasya, svapnaavabhodasya—regulated meals, recreation, work and sleep.

The reason why the Bhagwad Gita works is that its messages are timeless.

It's not about eating protein or avoiding carbs or fat but truly about realising one's potential and making the most out of one's life. Not about fitting into an XS size but taking the large opportunities that life throws at us.

Diet atyachar

Diet stories never fail to totally shock me. The latest one i heard: eat as much chewing gum as you want but don't eat food. Now why would somebody do this kind of diet atyachar? For results, of course. The result? Weight loss, my dear. And may i add—'guaranteed'.

Only eating biscuits that are 'low-fat' and have 'added fibre', replacing sugar with sweeteners, dinners that are just soup and salad, gulping down juices, smoking endlessly, twelve cups of coffee a day, Atkins, South Beach, cabbage soup—what is it within us that makes us 'try everything under the sun'? Why is it that we fail to use good old common sense when it comes to our body and health?

This disbelief in a common sense approach to getting fitter or losing weight persists despite repeated experiences (first- and second-hand) of crashing weight in no time and gaining double the weight in much shorter time than this 'no time'. Is it really so difficult to believe that a healthy lifestyle—which includes workouts, eating right and at the right time, regular wake-up and bed times—will help us lose our excessive fat stores and also help us get fitter, healthier and smarter? The obsession with Kareena's size zero is only a reflection of our perverted minds. The focus, if at all, should be on what she changed in her mind, eating habits, sleeping hours, etc. that brought about the change in her body, and not the body itself or its size.

Yoga and Ayurveda, the two traditional Indian systems, think of the body only as an ever-changing exterior of the very core of our being. Western scientists too have long woken up to the fact that the mind and body are interlinked. Though, of course, to understand that a calm, content state of mind leads to a healthy and lean body is not rocket science.

A mind which enjoys its share of peace realises that it has this basic responsibility of feeding its stomach at regular intervals. We also have an intrinsic sense which tells us when to eat and how much. We have all woken up in the night wailing as little infants, forcing our tired and sleep-deprived mothers to feed us. It's this regular eating pattern that protected us from infections, improved our immunity and memory, sharpened our senses and learning skills, and developed our bones, tissues, organs and limbs. And the most important thing that it did was make us feel loved, protected and important.

Excessive fat stores are our body's way of coping with the condition of starvation that we put it through. We do this by keeping long gaps between our meals (lunch at 1 p.m., dinner at 10 p.m., nothing other than some tea/coffee in between) or by going on deprivation diets. If eating regularly is a way to nourish and love our body, not eating for long hours or depriving it of any 'real food' is a way of punishing it.

Our lifestyles are abusive enough. We really shouldn't be abusing our body any further in the name of dieting or losing weight. Weight loss that beats common sense or that which is brought about by depriving your body of carbs, fat or protein is the beginning of the end. The end of health, vitality and peace.

Food trends come and go and leave behind a history of fat people!

Interestingly, these trends appear to make us thinner than what we are—it's just that it never works like that. Someone said of data analytics that you have to look at the past to know what is coming in the future. It's the same with food trends. The game changer in any diet is what the latest villain gets replaced with. Fat was the villain in the 1970s; it got replaced with sugar and low-fat products flooded the market. Today sugar or carbs is the villain and fat is gaining newfound glory. Soon the villain is going to be protein—veganism is proof. Time and again, modern nutrition history has shown us that when you make a villain out of a food product, thirty years later it comes back as the hero, and what replaces it becomes the new villain. But as a population that would rather lose weight yesterday than make lifestyle changes today, learning—whether from the past or present—for a better future or at least for a better body composition is asking for too much.

Let's look at three food trends:

1. Cold-pressed juices

Any box that you can open for detox, cleansing, fat burn, etc., is a wonderful revenue model and gets the cash registers ringing. It takes more than a beautiful revenue model to give you detox/cleanse/fat loss though. You need to open your heart and think—how fresh is this kale/apple/beetroot, etc. in my 'fresh juice'? All of us who are gifted with gums and teeth can just make the cold-pressed juice in our own mouth. That's when it really works wonders. Eating a whole fruit would also mean that you take the pains to actually visit the market and pick the fresh fruit or seasonal vegetable yourself. That way, even the main ingredient's purity, freshness, wholesomeness is guaranteed.

It's also about how you sell an idea. The good old aamras never got sold to us as cold-pressed, hand-crafted, polyphenols- and fibre-enriched, so we treat it with suspicion and link it to obesity. Not fair! We had it purely for its heavenly taste, and that's the fool-proof way to eat a fruit.

2. Paleo diet (presumably what early humans ate: meat, fish, vegetables and fruit, and excluding anything cultivated, like grains)

India, China and other ancient, and therefore more evolved, civilisations, have grown and celebrated rice for ages (Mohenjo-Daro had a flourishing trade in grains). Both India and China offer rice even to the dead, so if you are born into this DNA and gene pool, doubt you can escape it.

As for Paleo, it allows nuts, which are just like grains, cultivated, not exactly growing in the wild. The 'game' meat is not hunted with boulders and arrows but bought from a counter. So the risk of the genes interacting with the new environment is still very much prevalent. And then what about those grain-free muffins, protein-rich cookies and so on? Did the hunter-gatherer breed also make time to bake while living in their caves? For a culture like ours, which doesn't open boxes for breakfast or get 'take-out' for lunch/dinner, the meat-based diet is not 'wilder' or coarser than what we are currently eating. Also, making a villain out of any food group invariably leads to health issues, the carb-fever in the case of Paleo (where the body suffers from mild fever to full-blown adrenal fatigue and hormonal imbalance).

So i guess one needs to look at our ancestors in totality, give them more credit than being just hunters and gatherers and not overlook the value of eating wholesome, local and home-cooked, irrespective of where one lives.

3. Grow your own food

But everything is not so bleak: the hottest trend in food is the return of common sense. There is a—albeit tiny and slowly growing—population of the been-there-done-that, hotshot NY banker/rich socialite/not taking a job post IIM variety that's taking to farming. Real, hands-on farming. It's like the old left which respects the fact that it is capitalism that has afforded them the opportunity to farm. The good thing is that they are growing their own food, bartering it within their community and even selling it to those who will pay their price.

From haldi to curry patta, rice to mango, dudhi to drumstick, they are growing it with pride and selling it with a halo. More power to this variety. i hope their numbers increase and that it leads to India owning its mangoes and bananas with pride and not gushing over the blueberries and kiwi. It will also be nice if this trend leads to the use of native or heirloom seeds to grow more indigenous species versus going for the modified higher-yield variety.

Low on energy, high on marketed ignorance

The single biggest achievement of the weight-loss industry is the 'low carb-high protein' diktat. This mother of all myths can explain most of the food fads going around. But it is so well-entrenched in popular culture worldwide, propagated as it is by doctors, dietitians and trainers alike, that it has become a statement most of us don't even consider challenging. The most common ways in which it manifests itself are: Eating grilled chicken/fish/vegetables instead of the tastier cooked versions. Avoiding rice and roti for dinner and having just dal and sabzi instead. A thumbs-down to local fruits like mango, sitaphal or chickoo; only imported/exotic/supposedly low-cal ones instead. Multigrain bread, high-fibre, low-cal biscuits over regular ones. Avoiding sugar like the plague.

Our rich food and wellness traditions, as old as our civilisation, but unfortunately not well-documented and marketed, consider food as a blessing and not an entity to be broken down into carbs, proteins and fats. Not because they didn't have the labs to do so, but because they had the wisdom to understand that what matters is not what you eat, but how much of it is digested, absorbed, assimilated and excreted by the body. And food that tastes good is the only sure-shot way to deliver all its nutrients to the body. And what tastes good? Rice with dal and ghee, dosa with chutney, paratha with malai or curd, meat in gravy or biriyani—our traditional food combinations. But wait, this is something we know; it's right in our kitchens and it's for free, so it can't be valuable, right? Surely the labs testing things on mice in fancy places know better. It is 'research', after all. It must be for my benefit and not the corporations who will be selling those products.

Vegan or keto?

Recently, a headline declared that research has now proven that eating meat is not dangerous to health and that all these years we have been misled. They had looked at the same data as the studies which said limit meat intake and found their results to be statistically irrelevant. The keto community felt vindicated. On the other hand, the vegan community had lots to cheer about too. The documentary *The Game Changers* was successfully converting once hard-core meat-eaters to plant-based diets. Virat Kohli even tweeted about how he felt much better being a vegetarian athlete.

It's really not about meat but eating it in a sustainable manner without it taking a toll on our body or the planet. So, if you are from a traditional meat-eating community, go back to the practice of eating meat sometimes, two to three times a week max, and with rice or bhakri and sabzis, just like your grandmom taught you to. And if you are a vegetarian, don't worry about protein, just eat your dals and pulses with rice and bhakris and sabzis, just like your grandmom taught you to.

Carbs: friends, not enemies

i've learnt, over time, to diplomatically say nothing when someone tells me they are 'off carbs'. But keeping quiet doesn't seem to help, not with so many people succumbing to the 'no carbs' school of dieting. So here's another stab at demystifying—and yes, trashing—the 'avoid carbs at all costs' theory. First, some short answers: Are carbohydrates bad? No. Should i avoid them? No. How about not eating carbs for dinner? Bad idea. Carbs consist of carbon, hydrogen and oxygen in a continuous dance with each other. Depending on how loosely or closely they are tied to each other, we classify carbs as simple or complex. And we need both. You will find carbs in all fruits (simple), in all grains, dals and lentils (complex) and in all processed foods like cakes, biscuits, pizza, breads, ice creams, chocolates (not so complex, i.e., fibre-stripped grains and lots of sugar). The carbs we need to restrict are the processed ones. Why? Because they come with their share of trans-fats, sodium, preservatives, added colours and emulsifiers. They clog arteries, raise blood pressure, lead to mood swings and, of course, a bulging waist line. So, restrict such treats to once a week, preferably before sunset, when your digestive system is still in 'eat mode'. Grains like rice, wheat, jowar, ragi, bajra, and dals, lentils and fruits provide our body not just with energy-giving carbs but also with essential fatty acids, amino acids, fibre, B vitamins, micro minerals like selenium, zinc, chromium and many other nutrients. Taken together, they are anti-ageing, help lower blood pressure, increase peristalsis, improve fat-burning, lead to a slimmer waistline and a healthier heart. Further, when you eat roti with sabzi and dal, you improve both nutrient delivery and absorption. Avoiding carbs reduces your body's ability to burn fat.

The essence of fasting

While everything is turbulent and unpredictable, there is one thing that is constant, the shraddha or devotion to the higher reality. And hopefully with that the realisation of all that is impermanent. Bhasmantam shareeram—eventually the body is reduced to ashes. As the land of yoga, intellectually at least, we all buy into that. But emotionally, the attachment to the body is strong. And what i can tell you is whether it's Ramzan, Navratri or Paryushan, my inbox is flooded with 'what can i do to lose weight during this time' messages. Iss hamam mein, hum sab nange hai.

The purpose of every fast, drawing inspiration from the Covid-19 times, is to 'go inside'. Fasting, in fact, is about rethinking everything that consumes us, be it the obsession with weight loss, the body or the food we eat. Here's an attempt to put the practice of fasting into perspective.

The four pillars of a fast:

1. Swadhyaya—study of the self. It was meant as a practice that honed the mind, body and senses, to go inside, to connect with the formless, nameless, genderless, all pervasive life-force. And sorry to break your heart (and cultural appropriation by weight-loss industry), but no fast was meant for detox, cleanse, weight loss, etc. Which is why in Sanskrit it's called as upa-vaas, being in proximity to the supreme being, and is not called by a term that translates into guaranteed weight loss.

2. Tapa—voluntary renunciation (of certain foods for example). It was meant as a practice of introducing diversity to one's diet. To appreciate all that nature offers as food and to understand that health and harmony come from diversity. So if Lent encouraged followers to go meat-free and include more veggies in the diet, then

Paryushan brought millets and pulses into the spotlight by removing green veggies from the plate. Navratri or Ekadashi emphasised on tubers like suran, arbi, millets like rajgeera, etc., with generous offerings of nuts. And Ramzan on dates, fresh fruits and homemade milkshakes. Diversity is the key here, not deprivation.

3. Maitri—friendship and celebration: of the change in season, rituals and family bonds. Essentially a practice that allowed you to understand that variety is the spice of life. The fast didn't come randomly but followed a calendar that was based in deeper understanding. The fast wasn't a punishment for being fat but a celebration of life, a party to which everyone is invited and no one is shunned. The celebratory meals were and are for everyone, the ones who fast and the ones who don't. The ones who believe and the ones who don't. No one gets a lecture on fasting at the celebrations, just goaded to eat more.

4. Karuna—compassion. Any grandmother who follows roza will tell you that it is a reminder that no one should go hungry, and hence the practice of anna dana on almost a daily basis during Ramzan. In fact, irrespective of the name or the origin of the fast, if one developed a headache, nausea, weakness, it wasn't an endorsement of the effectiveness of the practice (wow, toxins are coming out) or something that one must endure but an indication that the fast must be stopped and normal routine should be resumed. Which is also why the very old, the very young, the pregnant, the ailing, women on periods, lactating mothers, etc., were discouraged from fasting. The idea was to be sensitive to pain and to

understand it, not to endure it. And to lead a life where one doesn't cause pain to oneself or others around.

Once you understand the essence of fasting, you will learn to value your body and will be able to drop the baggage of weight loss that you have been lugging around.

P.S.: *Hatha Yoga Pradipika*, one of the guiding texts of yoga, says that anyone on the path of yoga should stay away from all extremes, including fasting.

The joy of eating

Remember the last time you had a pastry, gulab jamun or pizza without guilt pangs? Most of us wouldn't, and if we did, that was probably when we were kids, all excited about birthday parties and cakes. (Did you know, all that anticipation actually makes it easier for the body to digest food?) But as we grow past the teens, we tend to associate food with fear and guilt. We become conscious about our bodies and can go to any extreme—starve ourselves or go on a crash diet—to 'stay in shape'.

Starving is commonly propagated as 'detox' or 'fasting' and is rampantly used as a weight-loss technique. Of course, fasting is powerful (Anna Hazare proved that), but as a means to lose weight, it's disastrous. As a method to shed pounds, it eats into all-important lean tissue that your body tries to hold on to.

When we starve, our body readjusts its metabolic rate to match the lowered or close-to-zero calorie intake. It does this by reducing BMR or basal metabolic rate, the exact opposite of which one should strive for to lose weight and stay fit. This is the 'starvation mode', where the body has already smartened up and reworked its daily calorie expenditure to carry on its basic functions, making you fatter in the bargain. (Muscle is the fuel, not fat.)

Ironically, the body does not come out of starvation mode as swiftly as it gets into it. Even after you start eating or consuming calories or break your fast, your body keeps working at a lowered metabolic rate. To make things worse, it also converts more calories to fat stores to prepare for the next fast.

The end result is often a frustrated mind and a body tired of trying to lose weight. The only way out is to eat in moderation and exercise regularly. All shortcuts, including fasting, are simply distractions.

The myth of detox—FAQs

Q: What is a detox diet?
A sham. It's a method of 'almost starvation' followed by people who are guilty of bingeing during Diwali or any other festival.

Q: Is going on a detox diet post Diwali a good option?
Detoxing during Diwali is a much better option. Traditionally, Diwali is all about detox. You detox your house by going into cleaning mode, letting go of things that you haven't used or don't work. You buy new curtains, cutlery, clothes; you give yourself a long, warm bath with medicinal herbs, etc. So with our mind, we should let go of 'guilt and punishment', they are useless, and instead bring in 'compassion and kindness'. It's

absolutely fine to eat sweets and fried food during Diwali. It's best to enjoy it in quantities you will be comfortable with so that you don't feel stuffed in your stomach and guilty in your head.

Q: Any quick detox recipes that have worked for your clients?

Eating food that is fresh and prepared with love is what has worked wonders for my clients.

Q: Do you recommend your clients to go on a detox diet after festivals/occasions when they are likely to overindulge in food that may not be appropriate for their bodies?

My clients are always eating right and their diets always include food that they love and relish. Indulgence, the way we understand it, is something that follows long periods of deprivation. So it's important to not deprive yourself and have an inclusive diet. A diet which includes all your favourite foods and lets you celebrate festivals without losing their true essence works well for everybody.

Q: Any celebrity clients who have gone on a detox diet suggested by you and achieved fantastic results.

My clients, including the celebs, work on having regular bedtime and waking-up hours, work out regularly, eat fresh and eat with a calm state of mind. Their stomach, body and mind is always feeling loved and nourished and the effects are for everybody to see. Cleansing the mind and body is a lifelong commitment, not a three- or seven-day detox plan.

Gluten-free and diabesity

The beautiful wheat fields in the fertile soil of the north Indian plains. For a few years now, the gluten-free craze has threatened the survival of this carefully planned crop cycle and the livelihood of the farmers.

While they never gave up on their rotis, parathas and their offering of kada prasad to the Gods, the urban folk found a new reason to blame their bloating, obesity and diabetes on gluten, the tiny little amino acid found in wheat. They quickly changed the type of cupcakes, breads and pizzas they were consuming to the gluten-free variety, paid five times more for it, and even introduced a little known cereal from South America—quinoa—into their diets. That it disturbed the ecology in its native countries and deprived the poor of their local grain didn't matter.

Science, as usual, has come around; it may be a few steps behind common sense and time-tested wisdom, but it always catches up. By 2013 we already knew that people who had avoided gluten in the last five years were fatter than the ones who had eaten it. By 2017, we knew that going gluten-free increases the risk to chronic inflammation, Type-2 Diabetes along with obesity (diabesity), the exact same conditions for which you avoided it in the first place. Hopefully, we will listen to both our inner voice and scientific wisdom, give up looking for health in packets and hashtags, and embrace a life of eating and cooking according to the region, season and genetics.

Good health is like success—there are no shortcuts to it.

Don't be fibre-fooled

Are you adding fibre to your khichdi, chapattis, biscuits or cereals? Think a little before you do that. Is fibre good? Yes, it is. But will it help you reduce your body fat, improve your metabolism, prevent diabetes, cholesterol, blood pressure problems and heart disease, as the glib marketers claim? Hmmm ... The truth is, all metabolic disorders or obesity-related conditions are based on more than one factor. Some of these are: food, exercise, sleep, relationships, genetics and lifestyle stress. So be it cholesterol, diabetes or reducing body fat, adding fibre to your life without addressing these problems won't get you anywhere. In fact, it may take you even closer to the disease that you're worried about.

Fibre is integral to digesting meals well, assimilating nutrients and excreting waste products. But it's best to encounter it through foods that naturally contain it, such as grains, pulses, sprouts, vegetables, fruits, rather than adding dollops of extra fibre to your atta. My one big reason for saying that is: zinc. Zinc is a micronutrient our body needs. It plays a critical role in synthesising the Insulin Degrading Enzyme (IDE), which keeps our insulin in balance. Adding excessive amounts of fibre to our meals reduces our ability to absorb zinc and synthesise IDE. Often it is the very people to whom fibre is aggressively marketed for its claimed health benefits who need to worry about their insulin levels; they suffer from a condition called hyperinsulinemia, commonly associated with diabetes and weight gain. So eat fibre-rich foods, they are good for you—but stay clear of fibre 'enriched' breads and cereals. As for biscuits, eat the ones you love, rather than the fibre-enriched ones that you think are 'healthier'. And remember: If you really want to lose weight, you shouldn't be eating biscuits at all.

Why you shouldn't have jeera, cinnamon, methi, haldi shots

Traditional cuisines are critical to good health because they use the therapeutic seeds, leaves, spices, fruits and vegetables in proportions and preparations that are time-tested. The fine line between use and abuse is crossed by overuse.

What's good as a part of a wholesome diet doesn't become a genie when trapped in a bottle.

Say NO to shots of cinnamon, jeera, methi, haldi, etc., and instead have them as part of your meals. If you want to get their full benefits.

Making The
Right Diet Choice

Rujuta Diwekar

Video link - bit.ly/rightdietchoice

UNSUSTAINABLE DIETS

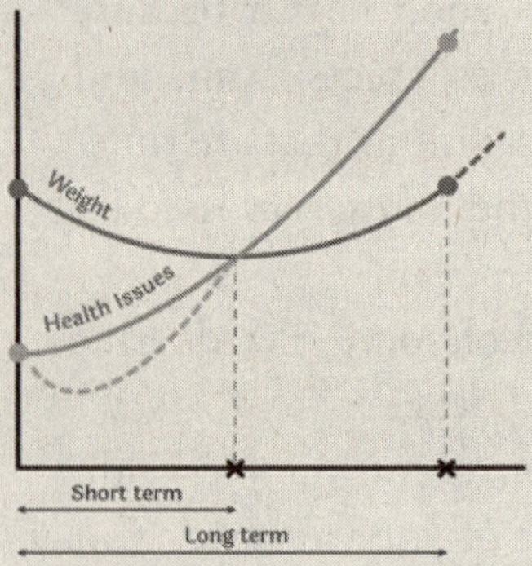

- In short term, you lose weight, but at the cost of health.
- Due to the placebo effect, you may mistakenly believe that health is improving.
- In long term, the weight comes back, and this time with many more health issues.

- Focus on carbs/proteins/ fats/calories.
- Deprivation of food groups or calories.
- Examples - Keto, LCHF, Paleo, IF, Atkins, etc. Always comes with a name
- Arbitrary rules - skip meals, eat non-traditional meals, calorie deficit, compensation diet, count macros.

SUSTAINABLE DIETS

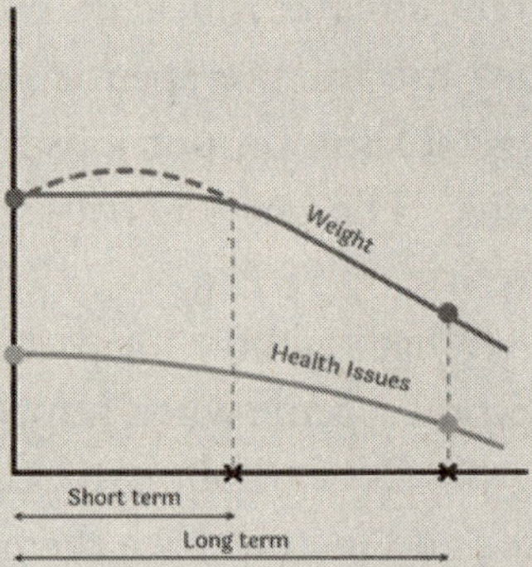

- In short term, you might not see a weight loss, but health starts to improve.
- In fact there could be an increase in total weight, due to increase in lean body weight.
- In long term, weight reduces and health improves consistently and irreversibly.

- Focus on local/ seasonal/ traditional.
- No deprivation, intuitive eating.
- Examples - home cooked food, seasonal specialties, traditional cooking methods.
- Common sense rules - no long meal gaps, eat slowly and without distractions, time tested meal combos and proportions.

Section Two

FOOD IS LOCAL, SEASONAL, TRADITIONAL

RUJUTA SAYS...

This Diwali, may our common sense shine bright and may we realise that sugar, salt or fat are not the problem, excesses are.

To the lord who made time during the war to expound on the values of eating and sleeping in the right amount, not too much, not too little. #Janmashtmi

May we strive to sacrifice our biases, prejudices and judgements today and every day. Eid Mubarak.

Holi is a yearly reminder that we need to focus on burning our fears, anxieties and lethargy and not calories.

The lord who dissolves all your creations so that you may constantly reinvent, restore and renew into a better you. #MahaShivratri.

May activity win over lethargy, fitness over weight loss, love over fear and finally our real selves over our lower selves. Happy Dassera!

2A. FESTIVAL FOODS

Diwali

When the ocean was churned, he emerged with the nectar of life, amrit, in his hands. With the message that the aspect of immortality of the self can only be realised through the health of the mortal self, the body.

Dhanvantari, the god of Ayurveda, generously imparts the lesson of eating according to the season, nurturing the forests and the native plants for the therapeutic value they add to our lives, and living in a state of harmony with our surroundings, to all those who pay attention.

Let the light of his teachings illuminate our lives with health, wellbeing and prosperity.

Diwali ki hardik shubhakamanaye!

Diwali foods and other myths

The best kinds of celebrations are those that focus on a festival's true essence, which in the case of Diwali, is all about giving and sharing. Excesses, unfortunately, are not limited to Diwali, Dussehra, Eid or Christmas—they are just more visible during festivals. Instead of focusing on the bingeing and guilt, these occasions have all the potential to become opportunities for us to fine-tune our daily life and return to the traditional ways of eating and cooking just like our grandmothers did. Festivals are a time to be grateful, not feel guilty for what you have on your plate, and to feast with a conscience.

1. Dieting and Diwali: The whole idea of being on a diet is to get healthier, fitter and leaner. If one must achieve that, then the diet must be one that is sustainable, and that means that it must be culture compliant. The ones that account for the big Diwali nights, morning pujas and the exchange of mithais and goodies. In fact, Diwali is a good time to figure if you are on a sustainable diet; if eating a regular Diwali meal amounts to breaking your diet, then it means that your weight-loss plans are going to be unsuccessful this time too.

Essentially, what this reveals is whether your diet fits into the game plan of the weight-loss industry. These unrealistic diets are not a culture fit; instead, they focus on the guilt around occasion-based feasting and take advantage of the same to sell detox plans or packages that are often extreme and doomed to fail.

A wholesome diet will teach you to eat without guilt and there really is nothing wrong in enjoying your pooris or halwa.

2. Preparing your body: Keep up with your regular exercise routine but bring it down a notch if you are staying awake till late. About five rounds of suryanamaskar will help you save on travel time to the gym, cost you less than fifteen minutes, leave you feeling fresh and can even help smoothen the digestive processes post bouts of overeating.

Regarding food, it's important to go back to grandma's basics; be grateful and not guilty for what you have on your plate, take only as much as you can finish and don't forget to share with the less fortunate while food is still fresh and hearts still warm.

Remember that there is no societal rule or religious ritual that requires us to only binge at odd hours, even if it is in keeping with the foolish belief that these chaotic meal timings make us seem young, carefree and cool. But clearly, no one looks cool or young while sporting paunches under flowing dresses, slouching on tables or burping during meals or waking up bloated the morning after.

Essentially, it's not the body but the entire lifestyle that needs to be prepared in the run-up to Diwali and even post that. i would love to sell you that dream of a fab bod in two weeks, but in reality, fitness is a compounding effect of small steps taken in the direction of health and harmony, every single day.

3. Mithai, the mistaken villain: There is an alternative to the fear of mithais—learn about their goodness and get educated about the basics. Let's not become a culture that replaces its Diwali goodies of kaju katri with dark chocolate, red velvet cupcakes or brownies, while the West is experimenting eating peanut bar or cashew crackle at some high-end cafe and washing it down with turmeric latte.

Ghee, one of the biggest components of most mithais, helps keep the intestines in good shape and ready to take on the load of overeating during Diwali. It is an essential fat and helps assimilate fat-soluble vitamins like A, D, E, K and therefore protects your bones, skin and immune function as the season changes. Sugar or jaggery is therapeutic when mixed with nuts, ghee, besan atta or gond (edible gum from the sap of the acacia tree) or sooji—all of which are nutrient-dense and delicious. Sweets made in ghee are a time-tested recipe that cause the least amount of disturbance to blood sugar levels. This fact is especially important to keep in mind for those who are diabetic or would like to lose weight.

Again, there are small things we can borrow from our collective wisdom, which are even more relevant today. For example, buy the besan from farms not malls to make laddoos. This will support the farmers who otherwise have to sell their pulses dirt cheap. Secondly, bring back the practice of making sweets at home. That is both a good workout and a lesson in gender equality, as it involves all the children, boy or girl. So, a good way to stay thin and raise sensitive boys and strong girls.

4. Dry fruits—good or bad?: Dry fruits are great when eaten the way they are meant to—first thing in the morning, as a snack or turned into a mithai. Nuts are an amazing source of amino acids, minerals and phytonutrients and all dry fruit is good: almonds, pistachio, cashew (it is a myth that the cashew nut is full of cholesterol; it has zero cholesterol and actually helps regulate it). The problem often lies in the form in which we consume it. For example, dried fruits are often eaten as chakhna (snacks) with alcoholic drinks, and that too in some ridiculous form like paneer tikka-flavoured cashews.

5. Diwali treats and sweets—choosing what to eat: For starters, avoid the packaged ones. They are often the low-grade variety picked up by someone with their bottom-line in mind and not your waistline or taste preferences. Instead, have homemade sweets and have them as part of

your lunch on any two days of the week. On the other days, you can have them as a snack between meals, a laddoo or a barfi at 4 p.m., or a portion of moong dal halwa at 6 p.m. when you are super hungry. Needless to say, avoid the low-sugar or low-fat variety—go for full-fat mithai.

Also, know that replacing sugar with stevia or any other sugar substitute, ghee with olive oil or fat-free cream, air frying instead of deep frying is not a healthier alternative. A homemade mithai eaten once a day over three to four days of the Diwali week won't land you in trouble. The actual game-changer in blood sugar regulation is really the late-night eating, so keep a lid on that instead.

6. A back-to-the-basics menu: The healthiest Diwali menu is one that sticks to the basics. It could be a simple spread comprising homemade mithai, one freshly fried item, one sabzi, one dal, some roti and rice, accompanied with some chutney, pickle or papad, and all of it served with love and attention to detail. Bring out your traditional silver thalis or kansa (bell metal) plates and have a leisurely sit-down dinner with conversations; indulge your guests with time and attention rather than an overwhelming variety of dishes. Break the monotony of heavy and multi-course Diwali meals with a touch of simple sophistication.

Quick tips for office and parties during Diwali

In office:

- Don't graze on the chocolates and cookies that may be kept around in canteens or lobbies as a part of the celebration.

• Instead, plan a day where colleagues bring a homemade mithai or savoury and eat it with all its glory, without the guilt.

• Direct the discussion towards the recipe, who in the family handed it down, is it a native dish of Gujarat or Madhya Pradesh and steer clear of nutrient- and calorie-based talks. Keep it simple and keep it interesting.

At parties:

• Eat a bit of dal-chawal or roti-sabzi or just a banana before you head out for a party.

• This will ensure that you have a sustained supply of glucose to your brain, which improves your chances of sticking to eating only those food items that appeal to you and only in amounts that don't leave you feeling dull and stuffed.

• Eat before you start drinking and have a glass of water between two drinks. This will ensure that you can hold your drink well and prevent a hangover the next day.

• If you reach home and feel some acidity, have a teaspoon of gulkand just before you go off to bed and first thing in the morning.

The post-Diwali detox

If your Diwali was accompanied by late nights, erratic mealtimes, etc., making you feel bloated and dull, here are the top three food items to help you recover:

1. Sugarcane: Chew on it or crush it fresh and drink its juice. India's traditional detox and go-to therapy for jaundice, sugarcane has properties to make you feel as good as new. Tulsi puja, which marks the end of Diwali,

has sugarcane as the main prasad for exactly this purpose: it allows you to detox from all the excesses of the festivities. It is rich in glycolic acid, the exact same thing that they use in expensive peels and cosmetics to bring back the glow on your face and even help restore the collagen tissue (bye-bye acne).

2. Tender coconut water: It can immediately fix the electrolyte balance and reduce bloating in the stomach. Definitely something that one must reach out for in the morning for a quick recovery from the late-night card parties. Don't forget to eat the tender coconut—the medium chain fatty acids in the coconut can boost your stamina and will actually help you feel energetic and not make you want to postpone your workout to the next morning.

3. Gulkand: Therapeutic mixture of rose petals, sugar and some herbs, gulkand can reduce and even prevent acidity. Excessive eating and sleep deprivation is a potent combo to ruin the gut flora and the intestinal mucus. Fortunately, something as tasty as gulkand is there to help. You can mix it in milk or simply have it by itself and it will put your intestines on the fast track to recovery.

And a special one: the mixture of one teaspoon of jaggery and ghee post lunch and dinner. Cleans up not just the intestines but sinuses too.

The case of shakkarpala

Diwali will be back year after year, but the shakkarpala is slowly but surely disappearing from our list of faral items. Once one of the supreme delicacies of Diwali, shakkarpala or shankarpala or shakkapada is now identified only as maida, and being health conscious means avoiding things with maida, so shankarpala, along with the chirota, is out. However, it's not the maida that's out, but these things:

- Family bonding: If not the rolling, the cutting of the shankarpala was invariably done by the kids of the household. Sitting on the floor, children cut out the nicely kneaded and rolled out atta into beautiful shapes. Squares, rectangles, rhomboids—maths finally had a tasty application in real life. And all this while listening to your mom and grandmom's stories of how they celebrated Diwali when they were young. Essentially it was a window to family history and of changing times.
- Gender equality: The fact that all the kids, regardless of gender, are involved sends out a message that kitchen activities are all-encompassing and that gender roles must be questioned. But it's done in a gentle way, one that doesn't involve conflict or confrontation and is a safe way to absorb a life-changing message.
- Economics: If not made at home, the shankarpala would come from small women's cooperatives or from the homes of underprivileged women who got the chance to make more money during the Diwali season. This money would often be used for their children's education, a small trip to the native village or were an extra deposit in the bank.
- Ecology: Since this meant family time together, no fuel would be burned to go to a mall or eat/buy things in there that come in non-biodegradable packaging. Shankarpala is born out of the collective wisdom of using

local ingredients and turning them into native meals, reducing the carbon footprint too. Wouldn't you agree?

i have avoided talking about the deep frying and the sugar, and that's because i have written about the glycaemic-index lowering properties of deep frying and the anti-ageing secret of sugar earlier. This post is to bring out the loss—the loss of traditions, economy, ecology and also health—that we suffer when we reduce food to one ingredient or nutrient. Food is all-encompassing and it's important to understand that if you want to leave behind a meaningful Diwali for generations to come. Otherwise, it will get limited to deals and shopping, and that will be truly, truly sad.

Harvest festivals

Gajak or pongal? Pick two!

Pongal, Makar Sankranti, Bihu, Lohri—from all corners of India, these harvest festivals seem to be giving us the exact same message: eat local, seasonal food to equip your bodies and mind to deal with the hard work that comes with the onset of the harvest season. Without adequate fuel or nutrients, the body will not be able to celebrate the opportunity to be active and instead will want to put the alarm on snooze. The main nutrient that these festivals celebrate is what modern nutrition calls 'essential fat'. Coconut, til, groundnuts, milk, ghee—each one of them is loaded with fats that are unique in their molecular structure, lending them an ability to allow the body to burn fat over other available fuels like carbs or protein.

Technically, the body is supposed to have unlimited stores of body fat that can be burned, and if we can use what sports nutrition calls an 'ergogenic aid', a nutrient which teaches or manipulates the body to burn more fat, we can see an increase in 'endurance performance', or stamina. So if you are one of those who complains about lethargy in the winter, who makes plans to work out but doesn't get out of bed, maybe all that you need is some therapy. And just because this therapy comes along with a celebration, is good to taste, melts in your mouth and doesn't have the seriousness and sadness of medicine doesn't make it any less potent. So bring on that chiki, gajak, laddoo, pongal and yes, have it exactly the way it is meant to be had—with joy, family, laughter and with generous doses of the other goodies.

Sankranti

Til gul ghya gaud gaud bola, amcha til-gul sandu naka, amchyashi kadhi bhandu naka. Literally translated—here take this sesame-jaggery ball and speak sweetly, don't drop it and never fight with me.

But i guess the hidden meaning is—don't ever drop the food traditions passed over from generations, i welcome you to experience the nutrients in local seeds, natural sugars and relish the sweetness of meaningful traditions.

Til or sesame is great for the health of bones, brain and the heart, thanks to its naturally high levels of phytosterol, fibre and copper. Sankranti, Bihu, Lohri, Pongal are all harvest festivals, ones that are filled with gratitude for the sun, weather and the farmer. On my recent trip to London, i saw huge til guls being sold in posh cafes as seed balls. Seeds are the new rage in the West and til is our indigenous produce, so it's heart-breaking when we turn to oats to lower cholesterol, and have almost stopped making til gul at home, sharing them and eating them together as a community.

May our lives be filled with the strength and sweetness of til gul.

Get rid of the confusion this Sankranti, and dig your teeth deep into the laddoo.

Holi

Thanda matlab 'thandai'

The colours of Holi are probably still on your face and hopefully you are staying away from the seasonal flu. Well, you would be if you had the traditional Holi meal—the one and only thandai—the spices, the herbs, the nuts and the milk with sugar.

Let's talk about sugar first. Boss, a can of cola has at least eight teaspoons of sugar and thandai will have barely one or two. So please, by any standard, whether diabetic, obese, heart disease, stress or whatever, you are in a safe zone to slurp up.

Now that that fear is taken care of, let's look at what really is the magic in thandai and why India traditionally has it during Holi, at the onset of summer, and how it prevents the heat from getting on your nerves. The clever use of almonds, khus-khus, pepper, cardamom, saffron and saunf makes for a really powerful energiser. One that uplifts your mood and allows you to ride smoothly over rough times. It restores your hormones to a state of balance. It is also rich in antioxidants, just that your grandmom didn't sell it to you on that peg. But most importantly, it's a great digestive aid, one that restores the mucus lining and gut-friendly bacteria.

And yes, it's great to taste too. So, though we are fed on a diet of 'thanda matlab', know that most of these drinks that claim to quench your thirst are dehydrating in nature. Not just the sugar but everything about them robs your body of the electrolyte balance. If you want the summer to be free of flatulence, acidity and bloating, you set that foundation with thandai.

Puran poli this Holi because

1. Thanks to chana dal, har bite mein fibre hai.
2. Thanks to ghee, har bite mein fat burning hai.
3. Thanks to atta and the combo with milk, har bite mein taste bhi, health bhi.

Bura na mano, bura mat bano, mazze karo—Holi hai!

The original organic colour for Holi—palash

The palash tree (Butea monosperma) is in full bloom and if you travel along the Mumbai–Ahmedabad highway, you will see it all over. A leafless tree, fully blooming with red-orange flowers, like a person in love who's lost herself but feels full of colour and cheer nevertheless.

No wonder then that this blooming tree was celebrated in ancient India as a form of Kamadev (God of love), agni (jawani ki garmi for us filmy types) and as a tree that whole-heartedly celebrates and declares the arrival of spring even in Tagore's poems.

The flowers are crushed to make Holi colour till date in rural and tribal India because we were cool long before the hashtag world of organic colours or safe Holi.

Gudi Padwa

If you have ever thought of detox, know that on Gudi Padwa, you chew on a few neem leaves so that all your systems are purified and ready for the shrikand poori.

Culturally, detox wasn't a punishment that followed celebration. Very simply, it was the connect to climate and crop cycle that paved the way for celebration.

May your detox ideas turn a new leaf this season.

Poori-shrikhand and how food combinations work

The summer will set in and the new year will start. It's a time to cleanse our thoughts, habits and rethink our belief system, that's what new starts are for.

With raging heat, the cow won't give as much milk, so this is the last time to make a delicacy out of a milk product till winter. As the temperatures soar, it is sugar that will allow the body to cool. When sugar is mixed with hung curd with its perfect combo of probiotic bacteria and essential fats, it doesn't load the pancreas. Shrikhand, when eaten with deep-fried poori, further ensures that glycaemic index of the meal stays low. As fat is important for a feeling of satiety, the chances of overeating are naturally low. A safe meal for all, including the ones struggling with obesity, diabetes or heart disease.

Ring in the new year with renewed glory, wash away your food fears and say a prayer of gratitude for the invisible masters of this delicious, clever poori-shrikhand and many similar regional food combinations.

Happy Gudi Padwa, happy Ugadi, happy new year.

Ramzan

An eating plan for Ramzan

Ramzan is a time for bhakti, devotion towards the supreme reality, and unconditional surrender of our ego and attachments (including attachment with food) through our prayers.

Roza is not limited to fasting; it's about overcoming temptation, and i think it's extremely important to remember that during iftaar. Since food is the most crucial and intimate part of our being, the way we consume food reflects our relationship with our innermost being. Iftaar is not some wild party where you eat to numb your hunger. It's a time to nurture your appetite with devotion and learn the importance of sharing, and so the common plate and prayers around it.

Below is a suggested framework for planning your meals during Ramzan. Remember, don't feast every evening in the lead up to Ramzan. Eat in peace and plan your meals in advance. Over-indulging in the evening or iftaar will not just dilute your concentration during prayers later but also leave you feeling gassy, bloated and constipated the next morning.

P.S.:

• The meal plan is more India-specific, so please feel free to include your local delicacies even if you don't see them in this plan.

• Adjust the number of meals as per your practice and local timings.

• Most of my Muslim clients across the globe will be following a similar eating pattern.

An eating plan for Ramzan

Rujuta Diwekar

(Modified for #Lockdown)

Meal timings	**Meal options**
Meal One (Saheri) On rising (within 10 mins) Before Fajar	Banana or any fresh fruit OR handful of dry fruits OR soaked black raisins OR Rice with milk Omelette + toast OR Bhakri/ roti + sabzi OR Roti + milk OR Paratha + curd OR Fruit yogurt (homemade) OR poha/ dosa /upma/ khakra OR pakhala/ choora &dahi
Meal Two Iftaar	Dates + Fresh fruit OR homemade fruit yogurt + glass of nimbu pani or chaas or kokam/bel/amla/ khus sherbet or gud ka paani or nannari (all homemade)
Meal Three Post Magrib	Homemade Poha or Seviyan or Dalia OR combos like - roti + sabzi + dal / rice + dal + sabzi/ rice + fish/ chicken + sabzi + roti/ veg pulao + raita/ rice with rajma or chole + dahi / paratha + dahi / khakra + moong / appam & stew/ dosai with veggies/ Moong dal khichdi & papad/ dahi rice / sabudana khichdi
Meal Four Post the big namaaz	Lassi OR Khichdi OR Protein shake OR glass of milk/ haldi milk OR paneer with veggies OR dahi & poha OR gulkand milk & sabja seeds
Bedtime	**Rub ghee to the soles of your feet**

Special tips:

Add:

- Milk to meals—will help you last longer without a drop in energy or hunger pangs.
- Ghee—to regulate blood sugars and to prevent overeating.
- Dahi—cools you down, restores electrolyte balance, prevents feelings of thirst.
- Soaked sabja—thermo-regulates, helps you avoid constipation.
- Gulkand—prevents acidity and bloating.
- Eat till you feel light not dull.

Workout:

- Don't work out with a stuffed or empty stomach.
- Best time is either just after big namaaz or sixty–ninety minutes after dinner post the big namaaz.
- Post-workout meal—within twenty minutes of the workout.
- Sip on water through the workout.
- Do not increase intensity or volume during Ramzan.
- Work at being consistent with exercise, it helps regulate your appetite.
- Work out in well-ventilated rooms to ensure a quick recovery.
- Pay attention to your warm-up and cool-down routines.
- Weight-training, yoga, sport, riding cycles, swimming, running, etc., as per your preference.
- Walking is an activity, walk through the day. Don't wait for post namaaz to walk.

Sleep:

- Stay gadget-free sixty minutes prior to bedtime.
- Regulate your bedtime.

Hydration:

- Avoid packaged juices/colas/store-brought sherbets.
- Check that urine is crystal clear, stay well hydrated.
- Not more than three cups of tea/coffee per day and not as the first or last thing in the day.
- Avoid packaged foods—bhujiya, chips, biscuits, ice cream, etc.

Narali purnima/ Raksha bandhan

On Narali purnima, which coincides with Raksha bandhan, coconut trees are planted along the coast as a bond of protection between land and water. By the looks of it, it's a pretty simple practice. As the monsoon starts, the fisher folk take a break for a couple of months and don't go out into the sea. Then, as the rains retreat, they get back to business as usual—and before doing so, offer a coconut to the sea along with a folk song and dance.

But if you take a deeper dive, you will discover how beautiful and well-thought out this festival is; it's a lesson about interdependence and partnership. Monsoon is the time when the fish breed and lay eggs, and if you fish now, you ruin the prospects of your business. Taking a break during this time not only makes economic sense, it is also ecologically sound, as overfishing and overexploitation are now well-documented threats to marine biodiversity and balance.

Native fishermen also intuitively knew what the latest research in nutrition science is now discovering: it's not about having omega 3s for heart health, it's about having a diverse diet. One that includes, amongst other things, essential fats from multiple sources, and therefore the break from eating fish and celebrating the coconut, a plant-based fat.

It's also the day to celebrate interdependence and the support system of having a sibling, celebrated with the rakhi—a thread of shared memories, responsibilities and resources. Today is also considered most auspicious to plant new trees, ones that will bear fruit, provide shade and become a home for birds and bees for generations to come.

P.S.: Narali purnima isn't just about serious life lessons: it is also a day of joy, celebration and good food. One of the specialties is coconut rice sweetened with sugar or jaggery and spiked with spices.

Paryushan, a celebration of pulses

Paryushan is the eight days of spirituality that Jains across the globe celebrate. The focus is on overcoming attachments, greed and fear, but Paryushan comes with its own dietary menu. No onions, garlic of course, but also no greens.

In a world obsessed with its green smoothies, this may seem out of tune, but scratch the surface and it's a whole new lesson in diversity and harmony.

While no green vegetables are allowed during these days, eating of pulses is strongly recommended. In fact, special preparations that involve a variety of pulses are cooked in Jain homes. Khichri, wadis, papads, you name it. It allows for a diverse variety of pulses to not just become a part of one's diet but also ensures a steady market demand for them, every year, and encourages farmers to continue planting native, forgotten pulses.

Pulses are so important for soil health that the UN had declared 2015 as the year of pulses to promote their farming. Pulses are so rich in amino acids (building blocks of protein), vitamins, minerals and fibre, that the latest Canada food guide of 2019 identifies it as both a vegetable and a protein source.

Essentially, we as Indians are living in interesting times. All our native practices are getting scientific validation from the West. But we must remember that the fine balance between man and nature doesn't come out of policies or recognition but intertwining food and culture.

Time and again, we must pause and reflect on our culture-crop-climate resilient way of life. And not trade it for short-lived trends or short-term gains.

Teej and sattu

Teej, a festival celebrated during shravan, is rooted in the concept of sustainability. It's the time of monsoon when a lot of communities don't eat fish/meat or green, leafy veggies like palak.

We still needed to get our folic acid, amino acids and minerals though, and therefore the invention of sattu. A delicious, intelligent mix of chana dal, gehu and rice flour (depending on the region you come from), it's the stuff that nutrition love stories are made of. #Plantbaseddiets as the US likes to call it, sattu provides the body with minerals like calcium, vitamins like folic acid and essential amino acids like lysine.

This is how sattu can help you:

- reduces menstrual cramps and clots.
- reduces dark circles under the eyes.
- reduces pigmentation and hair loss.

Diversity is an inbuilt system in our society and culture and it's time we own it with pride. Here's to Teej, sattu and all the beautiful women out there.

Janmashtami

White butter and why you must eat it

On Janmashtami, i woke up thinking if Krishna's mum Yashoda lived in 2019, would she be upset about her son stealing makhan or would she just worry that he was eating too much fat! Would she offer him a low-fat version? Or get his lipid profile checked?

Though the food of Gods, butter remains amongst the most misunderstood fats, along with milk and ghee. What's makhan? It's freshly churned butter from milk, an essential step before ghee. The churning itself makes the makhan special in terms of molecular gastronomy, not just in terms of its unique, 'melt in an instant' texture, but it also nutritionally equips it with many special properties.

For starters, it retains the potency of the fat-soluble vitamins A, D, K and E, therefore making it a powerful antioxidant. Then there is the Wulzen factor, a hormone-like substance only found in freshly churned butter that has the capacity to prevent joint stiffness and ensures that your bones store more calcium.

Freshly churned white butter is relished across India with regional delicacies that are fibre- and mineral-rich, mostly coarse grains and legumes, be it makai roti in Punjab, thalipeeth in Maharashtra, ragi adai in the south or namak chai (barley, salt and butter tea) in the Himalayas. The reason here is fibre and the glycosphingolipids, a type of fatty acid found in white butter, which works at protecting the gastrointestinal tract from infections or just from slowing down. Gassy, bloated, burpy? That spoonful of makhan may just do the trick for you.

Rishinchi bhaji

The makhan chor left behind a legacy of relishing one's meals. He truly believed in diversity of food and saw prasad (offering of food) as one of the forms of bhakti or devotion. Rishinchi bhaji (sage's vegetable) is one such delicacy cooked and relished on Janmashtami. It's a bhaji just with all the wild greens and makai, the harvest of the season, cooked in their own juices. It's best enjoyed with rice or jowar bhakri with a dollop of white butter or ghee and some dahi on the side. i also eat some alu wadi to go with it.

RECIPE OF RISHINCHI BHAJI

Ingredients:

Ghee
Green chillies, chopped
Red math deth
Ridge gourd
Lady finger
Red pumpkin
Sea salt
Buttermilk
Peanut powder
Cumin seeds
Colocasia leaves
Red math leaves
Snake gourd
Ghosale
Corn
Pinch of sugar
Grated fresh coconut

Steps:

- Heat the ghee in a pan, add cumin seeds.
- When the cumin starts to splutter, add the green chilli.
- Add all the vegetables. Sauté for some time.
- Cook well. You can cook this in pressure cooker also.
- Add sea salt, pinch of sugar and then the buttermilk (preferably buttermilk which we get when we make butter from curd).
- Finally, add the coconut and peanut powder.

Dahi and poha

Krishna enjoyed the dahi and poha offered by his friend Sudhama as much as he relished the chappan bhog (an offering of fifty-six dishes made especially on Janmashtami). Yogeshwar, as Krishna is often called, has a very simple message for all of us—without simplicity there can be no spirituality.

Pitrupaksh

It's the time of the year when you think about and thank your ancestors for all they did for you. It's because of them that the body is born and the body, the Upanishads believe, is born out of the food we eat.

Eating home food, with gratitude for the timeless wisdom of our ancestors who cooked using fresh ingredients, gently bringing out the best both in terms of taste and nourishment, is just one of the ways of thanking them and looking after our bodies.

When the physical body is endowed with health, spiritual growth begins to take root. It all boils down to what's on your plate and whether or not you have learnt to be grateful for it.

An eating plan for Navratri

The end of Pitrupaksh leads to the beginning of Navratri. Both, in their own way, use food or anna as a learning tool. Pitrupaksh is about charity and offering food to our ancestors who no longer live in their bodies and in the realm of our world. And Navratri, amongst many other things, is about staying disciplined with food to help nurture the creative and the feminine principle in our physical bodies.

Navratri is of special significance to women as they are live expressions of the divine mother. i believe it is our cultural or the Vedantic way of 'feminism', both fearless and joyful, in harmony with the dance of life. In a way, it teaches us that as women we must celebrate our lives every moment, and in every role we take up. Whether we choose to express ourselves as forms of Annapurna, Saraswati, Lakshmi, Durga, Kali, we are all beautiful.

Food is 'restricted' as a method to discipline the senses. It empowers the women with nutrients that make them not just physically stronger but helps bring about

Rujuta Diwekar

An eating plan for Navratri

Meal Timings	Meal options
Meal One- On rising	Fresh fruit/ Handful of nuts/ Overnight soaked raisins with kesar
Meal Two- Breakfast	Singhare ke pakode/ Sabudana khichdi/ Sweet potato with dahi/ Alu ki kheer/ Chana poori and halwa (on last day)
Meal Three- Lunch	Rajgira or kuttu or singhare atta ki roti with Alu or arbi sabzi/ Makhane ki sabzi or Kuttu ki kadhi with samo chaawal / upasacha thalipeeth
Meal Four - Dinner	Samo chawal with dahi / Jhangora kheer / Paneer ki sabzi with kuttu or singhare or rajgira or banana flour ki roti
Mid-meals	Fresh fruit/ Milkshake/ Chaas/ Shikanji/ kheer/ Shakarkandi ki chaat / Sabudana wada with dahi

Immediate benefits -

- Lesser mood swings
- Better hormonal balance
- Smoother digestion
- Clear skin and denser hair

a balance at the neuro-transmitter and hormonal level too. It's a 'religious' method of teaching families that the good physical health of the women and girls is of paramount importance to the wellbeing of communities and societies. It guides us to look after, nurture and create opportunities for women to express themselves freely versus suffocating them under the guise of 'culture', sabhyata or sanskriti.

This is a rough food plan but please make alterations to it based on the region you come from and according to what your grandmom approves :-).

Ganesh chaturthi

Don't miss the modaks!

As 'Ganapati Bappa Morya' echoes in the streets of Mumbai, 'Can i eat a modak?' is the question that echoes in the Mumbaikar's mind. Depending on the city you come from, the festival you celebrate and the mithai associated with it, similar questions would echo in your mind too. Weight-loss obsession hasn't taken away the sheen from our festivals, but it has surely managed to cast a dark cloud over our traditional desserts. Take the modak, for example. It's a traditional sweet made of rice dumplings filled with a coconut and jaggery mixture, sealed with ghee and steamed over boiling water, wrapped in a banana/turmeric leaf. Now, as the modak is made using local ingredients at home and it is delicious, it has all the virtues that make it 'fattening'. At least that's what the weight-loss industry tells us. i mean come on, it is, after all, not quinoa/acai berry/avocado!

Ganapati, who has a strong reputation as the Vighnaharta, or the remover of obstacles, loves the modak because he sees it as a nutrient-filled, antioxidant, fibre-rich, low-on-the-glycaemic index offering. The coconut and ghee provide a good combination of essential fats, just perfect to mobilise fatty acids from stubborn fat areas. The jaggery and rice combination works at steadying the blood sugars, ensuring a slow release of all the nutrients in your bloodstream and a calmer state of mind. The virtues of the modak, along with the therapeutic phytonutrients from the banana/turmeric leaf, don't get marketed in your face like the gluten-free cake. But they work for your digestion, health, weight loss—and the taste is pure bliss.

Modak, and why you must eat it

Devotee: because it is Bappa's favourite.
Constipated: because the ghee rebuilds the intestinal mucus lining and allows for smooth elimination of toxins.
Blood pressure: medium chain triglycerides in the coconut have a heart-protecting and BP-reducing effect
Cholesterol: the plant sterols found in coconut and the dry fruit stuffing helps reduce the LDL and improves HDL levels.
Diabetic: the rice, coconut, jaggery steamed, cooked and eaten with ghee is medium to low on the glycaemic index and completely SAFE, actually beneficial, for a steady blood sugar response.

Arthritis: the butyric acid found in ghee is a traditional therapy to reduce inflammation in every tissue of the body, more specifically in the joints.
PCOD: the rice flour helps in stabilising blood sugars and the vitamin B1 found in rice helps reduce PMS and sugar cravings.
Thyroid: celebrated as an anti-ageing mixture, this is one delicacy that your thyroid gland will thank you for.
Trying to lose weight: medium to low on the glycaemic index, full of good fat—nutritionally, there is just no reason for you to avoid it. In the scriptures, it is celebrated as a food for virya—means both vigour in the body and stability in the mind.
Ganapati Bappa Morya!!

Dussera

Dussera and the ten 'goods' of rice

One of our traditional festivals linked to the crop cycle, Dussera is when rice is harvested and looks like bars of gold laid out in the middle of the green fields.

Dussera also signifies the end of the ten heads that disconnect us from ourselves. Prejudice, fear, bias—we have seen it against rice too often, but since it's the day of good winning over evil, here's listing out the top ten 'goods' of rice.

1. Rice is a prebiotic, it feeds not just you but the diverse ecosystem of microbes within you.
2. Hand-milled, single-polished rice can be cooked in versatile ways from kanji to kheer and everything in between.

3. Leads to steady blood sugar response when you eat the way Indians (and native cultures across the globe) eat it—with pulses, dahi, kadhi, legumes, ghee, even meat. And yes, diabetics can eat rice too—there is no link between rice and metabolic syndrome (but if you keep believing it, you buy packets of oats and 'fibre-filled' biscuits, farms lose, food industry wins).
4. Easiest and lightest dinner meal ever. Leads to restorative sleep, which further leads to better hormonal balance. Especially required in the ageing and the very young.
5. Great for skin, gets rid of enlarged pores that come with high prolactin levels. Sustains and improves hair growth that an impaired thyroid may have damaged.
6. Rice-consuming societies are more gender equal.
7. You can make rangoli out of it.
8. Every part of the rice is usable, even the bran is fed to cattle.
9. Leaves behind adequate moisture in the soil to grow pulses, which then enrich the soil further by working as natural nitrogen fixtures.
10. Grandmom approved—local, seasonal, belongs to your food heritage. Sustains health, economy, ecology, PURE GOLD.

Annavaan bhavati
Dusserayacha hardik shubhecha
#riceisnice

Kada prasad on Guru Purab

If we go by the food and weight-loss industry, kada prasad shouldn't exist. At various points in your life, you must have come across the gluten-free, dairy-free, low-fat and sugar-is-poison trends. The food industry was always ready with alternatives though, profits over people is their motto after all. But kada prasad is still here and will continue to be.

Just like Guru Nanak and the essence of his teachings—staying strong and true to your beliefs against all odds and leading a label-free life.

Science as usual has come around, it may be a few steps behind common sense and time-tested wisdom, but it always catches up. This is what we know now:

- Going gluten free led to increased risk to chronic inflammation, Type-2 Diabetes along with obesity (diabesity), the exact same conditions for which you avoided it in the first place.
- Avoiding ghee led to an epidemic of Vitamin D-deficiency amongst many other issues.
- Avoiding sugar made from cane led to increased consumption of artificial sweeteners and the associated illnesses.

Hopefully we will listen to our inner voice, give up looking for health in packets, hashtags and labels and embrace a life of eating and cooking according to the region, season and tradition.

Ashadi Ekadashi

It's Ashadi Ekadashi and so my breakfast this morning was ratalyacha kees, a Marathi preparation made from sweet potato. With adequate help from ghee, curry patta, green chilli, jada namak and peanut powder.

Culturally, fasting was grandma's method of introducing diversity in daily diets. It wasn't about not eating, and that is something that people who fast for weight loss or even detox in the name of tradition often overlook. In fact, India has a vast array of what are known as 'fasting foods', so eating was very much on the agenda, just a little hatke.

It was about food stuff that offered a nutrient profile that your daily diet may fall short of. These turned into delicious preparations, often cooked using fresh ingredients of the season making their nutrients more available to the body than ever.

The sweet potato, for example, offers a rich supply of vitamin A. That way, you don't fall sick as the season changes. It also gives you some HMB, a metabolite of the essential amino acid, leucine. It's anti-catabolic in nature, so will arrest ageing, give you a toned body, prevent greying of hair, burn fat ... quite a gold mine there.

Need more reasons to eat traditional?

P.S.: Western countries are now adopting formal dietary guidelines to help their populations eat a more diverse diet.

Shila saptami

'Shila saptami' is the official break from cooking fresh, sanctioned by the planets and the moon. A day where you eat yesterday's bhakri (jowar/nachni/rice) with milk or curd so that your body is able to restore its water balance, rid itself of bloating and acidity. The 'shili' or stale bhakri is enriched with good bacteria because it's left untouched overnight. The milk, jaggery, ghee along with which it is had, further strengthens the gut health and is said to be one of India's ancient and well-preserved anti-ageing secrets. #Indianfoodwisdom

Kojagiri

Kojagiri is the night where you moon-bathe milk with dry fruits and rice flakes to keep the acidity down in the ever-changing weather. It keeps youth alive (jagrit) too :-). On Kojagiri, Lakshmi visits your home to bestow the wealth of youth, fertility and health. That's also the reason why Maharashtrians spend the night singing melodious tunes, all in celebration of youth, charm and romance :-).

“

RUJUTA SAYS...

This summer, be so cool that you flaunt your local fruit with pride!

Lemon grass in your chai to beat bloating and coughing this monsoon.

Rich in anti-ageing vitamins and enzymes, makhan (white butter) enhances not just the taste of food but life itself. The food of Gods!

Modaks filled with prayers, jaggery, coconut, covered in the soothing rice when eaten with hot ghee allows you to experience instant spirituality!

Navroz Mubarak! The much-needed reminder that sugar adds sweetness not just to our food but to our communities and to life itself!

Chew slowly, relish every bite and be grateful for the food on your plate—recipe for a healthy life.

”

2B. SEASONAL FOODS

i) Winter

The top five divine delicacies for winter

Whether it is health, economy or ecology, without sustainability, they lead nowhere. This is the indigenous thought behind all festivals and especially Tulsi vivah which marks the end of Diwali, and beginning of the cold season. Along with tulsi, there is all of the local, affordable produce of the season which is also worshipped. A reminder of how they contribute in the preservation of health, economy and ecology. These include:

1. Sugarcane: Our oldest detox food, rejuvenates the liver and keeps the skin glowing in the winter sun.
2. Ber: Strengthens the immune system (great for kids who fall sick frequently) and improves the diversity of our diet.
3. Chincha or tamarind: A great digestive, even the seeds make for a smashing drink when mixed with buttermilk. It even makes it to the UNFAO's list of Neglected and Underutilised Species (NUS).
4. Amla: The king of winters, fights infections—and even the evil eye ;-)—with its high levels of vitamin C. Have it by itself, or as chyawanprash, pickle sherbet or even a moramba.
5. Til gul: A winter delicacy with essential fatty acids to add chaar chand to the celebrations.

An open letter from gajak!

Hi! Namaste. Satsriakal. This is gajak speaking, i'm calling to ask why you haven't been eating me, or my cousin, til-and-gud chiki (or laddoo) this season. After all, aren't we here to boost your immune function so that you can deal better with chilling temperatures, fog and smog? Now, don't distract yourself (or me) by applying that chapstick on your dry lips. Try popping a piece of me into your mouth instead. Let me explain. i am seasonal for a reason. That's why Ayurveda recommends me, so does local culture and tradition. Haven't you noticed all festivals held around this time celebrate me? Why would you prefer that hot tomato soup instead? i can keep you warmer than any soup on earth, and i taste at least ten times better. Remember: what tastes better, gets absorbed and assimilated better. And i swear on God, i am loaded with nutrients. Sample this:

Til: It's the richest non-dairy source of calcium and is also rich in essential fats, copper, magnesium and zinc. Now you do know colder temperatures mean more painful joints and that's exactly why food containing til should be consumed. It has all it takes to keep your bones, tendons, joints and ligaments well-nourished, lubricated, supple and pain-free. The vitamin E in til will help your joints too, and keep your lips from chapping and skin from turning itchy and, along with til's iron and vitamin B stores, give your skin a reddish-pink glow.

Gud: It is unrefined sugar and less sweet than sugar, which is why it blends so well with til, giving gajak, and the til chiki or laddoo their unique taste. Still not convinced?

Okay, how's this? My til and gud combination can accelerate your metabolism and burn those fat stores. Ah, now i've got your attention. Come on, you're running out of time. The chill won't last forever.

A lap of gajar halwa

'My mother has made gajar halwa, what should i do?'

It's a national shame that gajar halwa is treated like some venom and packaged cereal as a weight-loss agent. Now why would your mother, and her mother, whose generation celebrated the advent of winter with a piping hot bowl of gajar halwa, peppered with kishmish, almonds and love, teach their offspring to cook and eat this? Was it to harm the wellbeing of the kin or to enhance it? i will allow you a wild guess. As winter sets in, colds, cough and upper chest infections rise and vitamin A (present in gajar, as you learnt in school) can help improve your immune system and prevent these. Also the milk, ghee, dry fruits are all carriers of good fat, and are rich in protein, vitamin D and calcium. So nanima knew that a good way to prevent these aches and pains in the joints during winter is to allow for better assimilation of amino acids (repair, recovery), vitamin D and calcium (thyroid health and denser bones). No, i'm not trying to reduce the great gajar halwa to 'nutrients', but just drawing your attention to the fact that food that is cooked with love, warmth and joy in your kitchen can be, and in fact always is, a hundred times healthier than cereals/biscuits/yoghurts parading around as 'health food'. The vitamin A and vitamin D in packets entices us but don't seem so magical when they come in home-cooked swad bhara recipes. Sad, isn't it?

Tricks up amla's sleeve

With winter, it's officially time for the amla—Indian gooseberry, if you want to glam it up. It's rich not just in vitamin C but also in its ability to keep the stomach calm. Amalaki is what it is called in Sanskrit, and it's celebrated for its anti-ageing properties. So if winter gives you a flaky scalp and scaly skin, you know what is missing in life, the ability of the body to restore its moisture. Or to keep it simple, you are not assimilating enough nourishment from the food you are eating. This dryness is associated with ageing in Ayurveda, and amla, with its phytonutrients, antioxidants and digestive enzymes, can do the trick.

It's not for nothing that amla is an essential part of chyawanprash, a heritage therapeutic preparation for winter, and also of the triphala. These keep your body moistened and do not let it dry out. It's also a mild laxative, so it will liberate you from waking up feeling really bloated and being constipated too.

North India, with its harsh weather, celebrates amla sherbet in winter. Another favourite recipe is to pickle or sun-dry amla and turn it into an inherent part of winter meals. It keeps the sweet tooth at bay and pregnant women with morning sickness will vouch for its magical effect on nausea. And before you go, here's another thing: when you sit all cooped up in the winter only to get a tingling sensation run down your thighs, calves and toes and don't know what to do, amla is the answer again, for it's the wonder fruit's iron, magnesium and vitamin B which soothe the nerves.

And remember—*Amla ka doz, har roz* (from the twelve-week fitness project 2020).

RECIPE FOR AMLA PICKLE

Ingredients:

Amla, 250 gms
Ambe halad, 100 gms
Rai, 1 small katori
Methi dana, ½ teaspoon
Garlic, 3–4 pods, chopped
Jaggery, 2 teaspoons
Sea salt, ½ katori
Mirchi powder, 2 teaspoons
1 lemon
Hing, ¼ teaspoon
Haldi powder, 1 teaspoon
Oil, 1 small katori

Steps:

- Boil water, put off the gas and place the amla in the pot for 10 minutes.
- Cut the amla and ambe halad into small pieces.
- Grind the rai.
- Fry the methi seeds in a little oil and powder it.
- Mix the amla, ambe halad, garlic, jaggery, rai powder, methi powder, salt, mirchi powder.
- Add lemon juice to the mixture.

• Heat oil in a small pan, add a few rai seeds, wait till it splutters, add hing and then haldi powder. Allow this to cool down to room temperature.

• Add to the mixture.

• Store in airtight glass bottle. It will be ready to eat after two days.

Note: You can also add ginger to this as a variation.

Also, instead of mirchi powder, you can use green chillies.

A bikini bod in wedding season!

In winter wedding madness, has vanity kissed sanity goodbye? Are those extensive five-day functions making you groggy, bloated, heavy, dull and lethargic the next day? Have you been loading your plate with more than you can handle (pun intended)?

Below are five ways to protect both yourself and your stomach from this atyachar:

• Most weddings are late-night affairs. By the time you get down to eating, it may already be 11 p.m. Have dinner at home an hour or two prior to leaving. This way, you won't overeat.

• Don't eat sweets and desserts at every party. Plan dessert days beforehand.

• Would it really be so bad to just say no? If anything, the look on your aunt's face will make for temporary amusement.

• Check out the buffet spread before grabbing a plate. Mentally note the food that interests you. Allow yourself two to three items and savour them.

The hair, skin and nails diet for winter

	How?	Why?	For NRIs
1. Dry coconut	Make laddoos, barfis, halwa or eat as a mid-meal/afternoon snack (dry coconut + jaggery). Can even add peanuts or chana to make it more wholesome.	—Essential fatty acids add lustre to hair, natural glow to face, prevent lips from chapping. —Micronutrient-dense, especially good for preventing split ends and dandruff.	—Desiccated coconut, coconut flour, coconut bread.
2. Gul (jaggery)	Mix with ghee and eat it with roti, add it to laddoo, use it as a mouth freshener.	—Digestive agent, will help get rid of dull nails or acne spots on face. —Good source of iron and other minerals, prevents pimples.	—Jaggery powders (darker is better), raw cane sugar.

	How?	Why?	For NRIs
3. Soonth (dry ginger)	—Dry ginger in milk/chai or laddoo or mixed with coconut (or til oil) and applied to scalp.	—Rich in antioxidants, prevents skin and hair damage. —The essential oils work as a natural hair conditioner.	—Add to chai, use it spice up your salad or pumpkin, squash soups.
4. Til (sesame)	—Laddoos and chikis or add til to your sabzi, dals and even rotis.	—Mineral-rich and great to keep the skin moist and fight pigmentation. —Vitamins B1 and E help nourish the scalp and prevent greying.	—Tahini on bread, sesame bread sticks, sesame bars/ crackles.
5. Rajgeera (amaranth)	—Roll it into a laddoo or chiki or make it into a roti.	—Rich in lysine, an amino acid that propels hair growth. —Folate bring shine to the skin and hair.	—Amaranth bars/ walnut amaranth breads.

• If there is a fourth—or fifth—item that tempts you, go close to the dish and whisper, 'Not tonight baby, i will make it up to you next time, i promise.'

ii) Summer

Hurda, poong and us

Last night i was at a hurda party. i know you don't know what hurda is—it isn't some exotic grain, crossing continents to land in the 'diet/health' food section. It is just the humble, local and unripe jowar. As the winter eases out and the summer sun makes an appearance, Gujarat eats poong and western Maharashtra eats hurda. Friends, families and kids all come together in a celebratory mood to eat them along with garlic, peanut, coconut and black pepper chutneys, and jaggery and curd. Sounds exotic, ha?

It tastes even better. Other than the natural feel-good hormones that meeting family and friends release, these hurda and poong parties serve a huge physiological purpose too. The immature grain is sweet to taste (will remind you of sweet corn) and is rich in protein, fibre and minerals. The chutneys and the curd make it easier for the body to assimilate the minerals, specially calcium and iron, without loading the gastro-intestinal system. Our joints and bones don't really feel up to the mark in winter, so to begin the summer season with a dose of amino acids, calcium and iron is just what the doctor ordered.

The only thing is it doesn't taste like medicine, it tastes yummy. So it's like getting an immune booster not just for yourself, but for friends, family and children. Whoever initiated this tradition had wisdom beyond the comprehension of modern nutrition science and dietitians. i mean, our poor health affects us, yes, but even when loved ones feel under the weather, it affects us. The hurda and the poong get-togethers are just one of the many rich traditions that India has had that maintain our health and improve our wellbeing. i pray that we don't lose our food traditions in our mad rush to lose weight.

Top ten summer foods

When summer arrives, the magazines are flooded with 'summer detox' and similar articles. But then most things we read will either be a rehash of what we read last year or stuff that just doesn't apply to our climate, temperament and palate. So here's re-introducing grandma's wisdom, or you could call it just common sense. It's the stuff that looks after the environment both outside and inside our system, it doesn't call for kiwis from New Zealand or quinoa from South America. It's about patronising our local farmers, relishing our home-grown recipes and, yes, eating food that makes you look as yummy as it tastes.

Here goes a top ten list:

1. Matka water: Bring back the matka, the malmal cloth and khus-khus grass; make it a centrepiece, in fact. Add the khus-khus grass to the bottom of the matka, pour water on top and wrap a malmal cloth around it. How does it help you? Well khus-khus is India's ancient

secret of keeping everything cool—yes our people knew how to make water thanda even before the advent of refrigerators. The porous matka adds a unique taste and keeps water free of any pathogens—let's call it pure and mineral-enriched. Let's call the khus-khus a herb, and there you have it—pure, mineral-rich and herb-infused water for a complete detox of the system. Well, if you had a business brain, you would be selling this water—anything in the name of detox works ;-). Khus-khus is also known as vetiver, and you will find it in all high-end soaps and perfumes, not just for its distinct aroma but for its ability to reduce emotional anxiety and bring about a calming effect.

2. Dahi: For all those who suffer from constipation, gas and acidity in the summer, this one is an absolute must-have on a daily basis. The thing, though, is that you must set the curd at home and with whole milk. This allows the essential fats, the vitamin D and the vitamin B along with the B12 to be retained. The process of turning milk into dahi naturally enhances the dahi with the 'good bacteria'. The growth of this essential bacteria is curtailed in the 'probiotic' products available in the market; that's exactly why they don't go bad for days together. Dahi will help make your intestines strong, reduce acidity attacks and keep the bloating down. For best results, have dahi-rice as a meal.

3. Gulkand: Another super food made with rose petals and sugar along with some traditional herbs and spices. Prevents breakouts on the face and keeps skin fresh and glowing all through the summer. It's another hidden

gem from the Indian kitchen—rich in phytonutrients, polyphenols and probiotics. So tasty that you will have trouble thinking of it as a therapeutic product. Start your day with a teaspoon or have half a teaspoon with lunch and dinner.

4. Kokum sherbet: Or Garcinia Indica, if you prefer exotic and non-local names. Native to the Western Ghats of India, kokum has been traditionally used as a fruit, as a part of curry and very popularly as a sherbet. Other than ensuring that no ulcer grows in your mouth or stomach during summer, it also works as an anti-obesity agent and most importantly has properties to prevent cancer. Little wonder then that it is bestowed with the status of 'amrut' or nectar in the native regions along the Konkan coast.

5. Sabja seeds: Move over chia seeds. Before the age of internet and the flood of weight-loss ads about chia, sabja seeds floated on every falooda, chaas and kheer in Indian homes. Not just a quick detox but an instant cooler and bloating reliever. Even a glass of water with soaked sabja seeds can help you get thinner—try it before you wear your favourite dress or before you step out in style for that party.

6. Mango: Before you want to strike it off your list, you must know that to look like a queen, you will need to keep good company of this king of fruits. Mango is great to taste, it's a quick and effective cleanser of the entire system and an under-utilised (in fact, most times misunderstood) weight-loss aid. Do soak it in water for about twenty–thirty minutes before consumption.

7. Nariyal pani: The divine nectar from the most divine fruit that India has to offer is not just a thirst-quencher but has the perfect balance of sodium and potassium required to give your skin a baby-fresh look. Yes, it prevents dehydration too and is a well-known cramp and migraine reliever during PMS trouble.

8. Jeera: You may not have thought much of this humble Indian spice, but it can detox your system, calm your nerves and aid your fat-burning efforts this summer. Roast it a bit and turn it into a powder, add it to your chaas with a pinch of kala namak, and you will feel and look cooler than ever.

9. Cashew apple: It's the conical fruit out of which the cashew nut sprouts. Five times richer in vitamin C than an orange, this one makes for a perfect tangy drink with just a single bite. That's exactly why even the global food giants are interested in it. Brazilians love this fruit and eat it not just for its detoxing properties but also for its ability to zing up your sex life and burn stubborn fat. Last word—don't ignore this local but exotic fruit.

10. Jowar: Jowar is one of India's ancient grains and is naturally cooling in nature. So if you really want to overcome that weight-loss plateau this summer, then bring jowar rotis or bhakris back on your plate. If you want it to work as a weight-loss aid, then be generous with the ghee you add to the jowar roti. Rich in vitamin B1, iron and fibre, it can help you pick up the rate at which the body is burning fat. It's also popular in India as a brain food. You want to look sleek and smart, go get jowar.

Khus

Say hello to khus roots, Mother Nature's natural coolants. They not only make your paani thanda but have exceptional health benefits especially in cases of hormonal disorders like PCOD and low sperm mobility.

Some other important benefits:

- smooth, flawless complexion.
- prevents UTI and fevers.
- relief from chronic body aches and pains.

Where to find it:

Grows all over India. It was earlier used in matkas to naturally cool down the water and give it a mild fragrance similar to chandan. The grass is used to make mats, curtains, chatais, especially in areas of dry heat, as it's known to make the room and surroundings cooler. It's often turned into a khas sherbet too.

Farmers grow it around veggies and fruit trees for its anti-termite and insect-repellent properties.

How to use:

Clean roots and soak them in your drinking water. You can keep them in for three days. Post that, remove them, dry them and reuse up to three times.

Also known as wala, walo, vetiver, ramacham.

Summer fruits to bite into

Wikipedia defines neglected and underused (NUS) crops as domesticated plant species that have been used for centuries or even millennia for their nutritional and medicinal properties but have been reduced in importance over time due to unrecognised nutritional value, poor awareness and reputational problems ('poor people's food'). These are some underused summer fruits and why you must have them.

Karvanda: This drought-resistant fruit that grows from the Western Ghats to Afghanistan can save you from a lot of the heartache that comes with constipation. Rich in micronutrients, it can strengthen the digestive system and pancreas, making it an effective medicine for diabetes. Folk medicine also celebrates it for its ability to reduce the chances of anaemia and increase haemoglobin levels, thereby helping in fertility.

Tadgola: Sometimes fancily called ice apple, the fruit of the toddy or sugar palm is literally a godsend. The hard exterior protects the fleshy, juicy fruit and you need some serious expertise in opening it without damaging the fruit or your hand. Celebrated as the perfect liver cleanser, this is *the* summer detox to look out for. And it helps control blood pressure.

Jamun: The Indian government has fought off attempts to patent it and turn it into medicine for diabetes, and luckily we can buy it at local markets for a steal. Great to taste, the polyphenols and micronutrients will not just keep blood sugars stable but help reduce effects of ageing too. Cultivated by local farmers, these are the fruits we should be promoting to ward off everything from constipation to BP, anaemia to diabetes. A small but effective step for farmers and local economy.

Panha

Bloated, tired and irritable in the heat? Try panha, raw mango sherbet—the potassium will cool you down and the enzymes will aid digestion.

High on tryptophan, an essential amino acid, mango is naturally rich in the nutrient you need to feel happy. Happy is healthy :-).

More summer drinks

Three drinks to uplift your spirits this summer:
1. Nimbu sherbet at mid-morning around 11 a.m.
2. Buttermilk (chaas/taak) with lunch.
3. Milk with gulkand at bedtime.

Special nimbu pani

Nimbu pani with kala namak, sugar, kesar and a bit of ginger works wonders as a mid-afternoon pick me up drink (couple of hours post lunch).
Tip: Keeps the afternoon slump away. The kesar works miracles for the hair and skin while the ginger and kala namak combo will leave you feeling light and helps avoid bloating on tough working days.

Chikodi: gift of the sun

Open the door of your mind and heart and allow the goodness of the chikodi to come in. It brings you the wisdom of your past, the labour of your grandmother and the blessings of the sun. These are small papads made from sabudana, a delicacy in Maharashtra.

This lockdown has made me wonder at the brilliance of our grandmoms. Their kitchens, cooking and life was pandemic-proof. They stored dals, grains, millets and spices for the full year. And also made papads from dals, vegetables, millets and even fruits (aam papad) in summer, which were then eaten during monsoon. (Not even counting the morambas and achaars here.)

This ensured that should there be an emergency or an unprecedented situation, there need not be a compromise on the taste or the goodness (nutrients if you like) that homemade meals have to offer.

Their lives were #wasteproof #futureproof #bakwasproof. Just so much to learn from the way they lived and so much to receive from what they have left behind. A treasure-trove of love, compassion and common sense.

RECIPE OF CHIKODI/CHIKVADYA

Ingredients:

Sago (sabudana), 1 katori
Water, 5 katoris
Cumin seeds, ¼ teaspoon
Salt

Steps:

- Wash the sabudana and leave it to soak overnight (there should be half-inch water above it so it soaks properly).
- In the morning, heat up five katoris of water.
- When the water starts boiling, add the sabudana and stir continuously till the mixture becomes sticky and transparent. (To check that the mixture is cooked properly, put one teaspoon of it on a plate—the mixture should not spread.)
- Add salt and cumin seeds. (Remember that, after drying, the salty taste increases).

- Now take a clean butter paper and place out teaspoons of the mixture on it, evenly spaced). Keep the paper in the hot sun.
- In the evening, remove from the paper, transfer to a thali and dry again for one–two days.
- Fry in oil whenever you want to eat it.

Chikvadya remain fresh and tasty for one year at least.

iii. Monsoon

The food guide for monsoon

Eating according to the season and region is the foundation of staying healthy. It allows individuals to have better health but also contributes towards the local economy and helps keep the global ecology in a state of balance. Here is a guide on what you can eat during monsoon:

1. Vegetables: The soil during the rains is not suitable to grow green, leafy vegetables and therefore we shift to creepers like doodhi, pumpkin, karela, gilka and root vegetables like sweet potato, suran and konfal. The exception to this rule are the wild and uncultivated greens that shoot up during the season—ambadi, shevla, lingdi, to name a few. Every region has its own, and special recipes to go with it. It's very important for your gut-bacterial diversity and acts as a booster shot for immunity.

2. Grains and millets: Nachni is the millet for rains. You can eat it as porridge, bhakri or even a papad. Say no to multigrain bread, attas and biscuits though. The season also comes with festivals and special months like Shravan, where the focus shifts to eating smaller millets like rajgeera, samo, kuttu, mandua, etc. Again, have them in traditional preps and in combination with dahi, makhan, etc., to ensure optimum assimilation. Note that rice, jowar and wheat can be eaten throughout the year. Also corn, but insist on desi corn and not sweet/American corn.

3. Pulses: Traditionally, as Indians went off meat/fish during the rains, the pulses that were carefully dried and segregated during summer would serve as the source of protein, vitamins, minerals and even fibre during this season. The best ones turn into usals, the next grade to dals, the one after that to wadis (that can be cooked as sabzi and is often a mix of many pulses) and papads. Zero-wastage policy has been an integral part of our culture. Two important pulses you must incorporate in your meals this season are kulith (horse gram) and alsaane (goa beans). Great for skin and hair. Please note that the Canada food guidelines now recognise pulses both as a vegetable and protein.

4. Specialty items: Every season has its own king, if it's mangoes for summer, then it's deep-fried bhajiya for the rains. Use filtered groundnut/mustard/coconut oils and don't re-use the oil for cooking afterwards. Remember that without essential fat in the diet, vitamin D cannot get assimilated, and that essential fats also help in regulating

blood sugar. So apart from being tasty, deep-fried pakodas are healthy too (and for everyone, heart patients, obese and diabetics included); eat them without fear and with the confidence that you know when to stop eating.

When fried are friends

Most of us romanticise about a lazy evening spent watching the pitter-patter of rain on our window along with pakoda and adrak chai. Ever wondered why? Here are two reasons:

We are facing an epidemic of vitamin D deficiency that is not just linked to obesity but to every lifestyle disease including arthritis, diabetes, heart disease and even cancer. We get enough vitamin D from sunshine but it must get converted to vitamin D3, the usable form for the human body. Vitamin D cannot be absorbed in the body in the absence of essential fat. In comes desi ghee, and groundnut, mustard or coconut oils. Once a week this season, fry your aloo/ajwain/onion, what have you, in besan batter. And provide your body with the much-needed essential fat for vitamin D assimilation. And don't worry, eating essential fat doesn't lead to high cholesterol. And besan has a good amount of phytosterol and fibre, the same stuff that oats have and sell themselves as cholesterol-lowering. Bite into the pakoda, it really is good for the heart!

The monsoon comes with its share of infections, fevers and other ailments. Your chances of falling sick are higher when your immunity is at its weakest. And one of the reasons why our immune system collapses is insufficient calorie intake. Your taste buds are not against your weight-loss plans, they are simply against your plan to lose your immunity. And to guard you against a possible crash of your immune system, it urges you to eat fried food. Essential fats, like in filtered groundnut oil, are rich in antioxidants that help you fight free radicals and prevent illness and also work at keeping your skin and scalp healthy (i am talking about the pakoda you make at home, where you don't reuse oil). And the reason you want an adrak chai with which to round off the pakodas is because ginger aids your intestines to break down fat and rids your stomach of gas. That way, you take care of overindulgence too.

What is the monsoon green in your region?

Even while green smoothies of broccoli, avocado, celery and the likes make a quick buck for the weight-loss industry, the shevla grows not more than fifty km from where you stay, but you say, what's shevla? And that's why, deviyon aur sajjano, we stay fat.

But then, what is shevla? It's a wild, uncultivated vegetable and grows just for a week or two as monsoon begins. You eat this as a seasonal specialty and as a bonus it will repair a leaky, weak gut, boost your immunity and give you a booster shot of vitamin B and micro-minerals.

P.S.: Eating non-local adds to climate change even if it's done in the name of vegan, keto or detox.

Frizzy hair? Split ends? Dry scalp? A simple DIY for hair health

Come rains, most of us will have one, or worse, all of the conditions above. Shampoo companies even make special ads to lure us into buying their products. But chill, Mother Nature has already sorted this stuff out for us.

There's vala (vetiver or khus roots), goonja seeds (rosary pea) and good old tulsi with its beej or seeds. You will find these at local farms and Ayurvedic stores across India. And here's the simple DIY for hair health:

1. Take a glass bottle with a broad bottom.
2. Put two–three roots, one–two tulsi stalks, one–two goonja seeds and put them in the bottle.
3. Pour coconut or mustard oil into the bottle and leave it to soak in the herbs for forty-eight hours.
4. Invite your friends or cousins over and give each other a good head, neck and shoulder massage.
5. Enjoy chai and bhajiya while at it, give duniya ko gaali and feel happy for having each other in this zaalim duniya. Also for having these wonderful herbs.
6. Leave the oil on overnight and wash. No need for conditioner. Use the weather and not the blower to dry.
7. Leave yourself impressed and find yourself so beautiful.

Try it and tell me how you feel.

And yes, it's great for hair fall too.

Top three foods to prevent hair loss this monsoon

1. Methi dana: Add it to some warm coconut oil, let it cool, then massage your scalp and leave overnight. Can also be added to kadhi and had with khichdi for dinner. Alternatively use it in tadka for veggies like pumpkin or to flavour your raita. The methi dana is especially useful if it's a hormonal issue-related hair loss (PCOD, etc.) as it helps improve insulin response.

2. Aliv seeds (garden cress, halim): Soak them in water for seven–eight hours and have them with milk in the night. Or roll these iron-rich seeds into laddoos with coconut and ghee for even better results. They also protect hair from loss that comes with chemo treatment.
3. Nutmeg: Add a small pinch to milk (along with aliv) and have it as a nightcap. The vitamin B6, folic acid and magnesium help de-stress and prevent hair loss.
Other ingredients that are useful:
Ghee—for its essential fats.
Haldi—for its immuno-boosting properties.
Dahi—for the minerals and probiotic bacteria.

For a glowing skin this monsoon—alu

This big, green, leafy vegetable is one of the many wild and uncultivated vegetables that grow during the rains. They are a treasure trove of micronutrients, especially the lesser-known ones like Hyaluronic Acid (HA). It's the stuff that most expensive derma products are made of. It gives your collagen and connective tissue a much needed boost and prevents all signs of ageing. And is known to give you a smooth, flawless, glowing complexion and even lustrous hair. HA even helps with vision issues, protects joints and is especially useful in rheumatoid arthritis.

These grow pan-India and are often used for their therapeutic purposes by our native folk. The name in Marathi is alu (not to be confused with potato) and the closest English name is colocasia.

Want to anti-age and look great? Ditch the mall and patronise the farm.

Here are some more reasons to eat alu:

1. Micro-minerals—food for hair fall and dandruff.
2. Fibre—good for digestion and bloating.
3. Zinc—good for pregnancy, foetal health and sex hormones.

Desi dates or fresh khajoor

- Improves haemoglobin levels.
- Used in treating sleep disorders—fights most infections and allergies.
- Boosts exercise performance—relief from constipation and acidity.

But the main reason why you should eat it is because it looks good, tastes good and is in season right now.

How can you eat it?

- First thing in the morning.
- Post lunch if Hb levels are low.
- Add to the kids' dabba, especially if they are around puberty.

Where can you buy?

- Local bazaars, and once you find it, save the seed and plant it in your compound.

Happy eating, people.

Chai in monsoon—three special tips

With the rains comes the desire to sit by the window, sipping a hot cup of chai. It surely calms your mind, but here are three easy tips to make it works for your body too.

1. Add ginger and tulsi—for digestion and immunity.
2. Add lemongrass—to prevent bloating and congestion.

3. Add black pepper or cinnamon—to improve insulin sensitivity.

FAQs on chai

1. When not to have chai/coffee:
• first thing on waking up.
• last thing before sleeping.
• in place of a meal during the day.
2. How many cups a day is okay?
Two–three cups are totally fine.
3. With sugar or sugar-free?
Add sugar to your chai/coffee, avoid the invisible sugar from packaged food (breakfast cereals, fruit juice, biscuits, etc.).

And have it with full-fat milk please.

Top three foods that you must eat in the month of Shravan

Shravan is the holiest month of the Hindu calendar. It's when the churning of the ocean and search for amrit took place. Legends aside, many wonder-foods are recommended in this month for the detoxification of the body. Here are the top three.

1. Banana flour: Traditionally used by people in coastal India to make adais, dosa, thalipeeths, even mithais. Food academics now recognise it as a prebiotic, which means it develops the infrastructure for your gut to retain the probiotic bacteria. Earlier sold only by small women's cooperatives, it now occupies space on health food counters as 'gluten free'. Made from sun-dried raw banana, it is used in heritage recipes to help the body store

more calcium. Good for all those with weak stomachs—from infants to seniors or those who have ruined their stomachs with crash dieting.

2. Peanuts: There isn't a single item that's used for upavas (fasts) that doesn't include peanuts. Rich in monounsaturated fats and resveratrol (the same nutrient that helped wine gain its heart-healthy reputation), it's known for its appetite-regulating properties. It is much needed, as it's easy for us to overeat sabudana khichdi and vadas. The next time you are going to a party where you fear you may overeat, just chew on a handful.

3. Coconut: Rich in the all-important fatty acid called lauric acid, coconut is known for its properties to provide the body with physical stamina and the mind with calm. Lauric acid, also found in human breast milk, is an antibacterial and anti-viral agent. Moreover, studies link coconut to a low waist-to-hip ratio, and coconut oil today is where virgin olive oil was a few years ago—the toast of every weight-loss diet.

RUJUTA SAYS...

Cooking is meditation with your eyes open.

What olive oil does to the Italian's heart, desi ghee does it to the desi heart. :-)

Kaha gaya common sense? When ghee in coffee is a multi-million dollar business and ghee with chawal a disappearing delicacy.

Some revolutionary stuff you can do today—eat dal-chawal for dinner, pay attention when someone talks to you and smile (not pout) for the camera.

Ragi/nachni is great for people who are anxious to lose weight. The amino acids help not just fat burning but are known to calm the mind too. Weight-loss nirvana. ;-)

It's not just a laddoo, it's an unbroken chain of love, wisdom and nourishment.

2C. DAILY SUPERFOODS

Superfoods and how to identify them

In the mad world of new superfoods every day, how do you identify the real from the unreal? Here are a few things you can look for:

1. Time-tested. Does your grandmom know it? Does she have multiple uses for it in her kitchen? Like the mango: a panha to cool you down, ambe dal to add flavour to your regular intake of amino acids, aamras with poori for celebrations, and achaar or loncha to accompany plain dahi-rice or dal-rice for the more sombre occasions.
2. Art. How does the artist community respond to that food? Is it on the border of a saree? The leaves on the entrance as a toran? Does it appear on tribal paintings? Is there a folk song, proverb, cultural anecdote or story for it?
3. People. Does it bring people together? Is it food for all? Does it unite us across the divide of class, gender, community, age? Does it bring happy memories? Does it ignite empathy in you? Does it inspire you to share or hoard?

Food is poorna bramha. Every tiny speck of anna holds within itself the power of the entire universe.

Long story short, patronise food that gives you the three E's: energy to your body, economy to your farmer, ecology to your globe.

Banana

Banana zaroor khana

1. Mood-booster
2. Fertility-booster
3. Immunity-booster
4. Digestive aid
5. Gut integrity-keeper
6. Hormone-regulator

Well, there are at least a dozen more reasons why you must eat the banana, in all its forms—kaccha, ripe, overripe and its flower.

But one of the best-kept secrets of an Indian kitchen is banana flour. Where raw bananas are skilfully peeled and then patiently sun-dried and crushed to make a flour. It's then turned into a thalipeeth or flat bread on an iron skillet and enjoyed with a freshly grated coconut chutney or a freshly pounded til chutney.

It's the kind of food that's fit for the goddess within. The shakti or the feminine power of action in every being.

RECIPE OF BANANA FLOUR THALIPEETH

Step 1: Prep of banana flour

- Remove the skin of the raw bananas.
- Cut horizontally to make ¼-inch pieces.
- Dry in the sun for two to three days.
- Grind to make flour.
- Store in an airtight glass bottle.
- You can use this as fasting food.

Step 2: Making thalipeeth

- Take one katori of the flour.
- Mix with one katori of smashed potatoes.
- Add green chillies, jeera powder (if you like), roasted peanut powder.
- Add water to make dough.
- Make small balls and spread over iron/cast iron tawa.
- Shallow fry using ghee.
- Serve with coconut chutney.

Banana flower

- Acne that leaves behind marks?
- Migraine that announces to the world that you are PMSing?
- Trying to get pregnant but period cycle not regulating?

Fikar not, the banana flower can help overcome it all.

The mineral-, vitamin-, flavonoids-rich banana flower is a brilliant and delicious way to improve insulin sensitivity. Especially useful for those with PCOS, endometriosis, diabetes. Eat the sabzi, usal, wadi once a week. Bye-bye bloating, irritability and all that.

Hair, skin and hormones—the magic of raw banana and boiled peanuts

If you would like the above in a state of balance and flourishing, eat this meal once every week: raw bananas cooked on a tava with oil, salt and seasoning as you like and boiled groundnuts with salt (add salt while boiling them).

• The resistant starch in bananas acts as a prebiotic and improves not just digestion but also blood sugar regulation.

• Boiled peanuts have an antioxidant profile that is even better than raw/roasted peanuts and that helps with the ageing effects on the skin.

• Together they ensure that you get a good dose of vitamin B6 which can cut down bloating and improve your mood.

• They also have minerals that are necessary for recovery processes of the body and for heart health.

• The monounsaturated fatty acids and vitamin E in peanuts and the antioxidants in the banana are especially useful for those who may have lost weight by crash-dieting or harsh procedures and are now seeing the ill-effects on the skin, hair and digestion.

• If you have endometriosis, painful PMS or high prolactin levels, make sure that you have both, the raw banana and boiled groundnuts, as a regular part of your food routine.

Jackfruit

Jack, fruit of all trades

And it's the time of the year when our tropical country produces one 'fattening' fruit after another—mango and then jackfruit. Fattening only according to someone's wild imagination though, as both these are zero in fat and cholesterol; they get a bad name simply because they are sweet.

Anyways, this column is a tribute to my favouritest fruit, the magical, delicious jackfruit. First things first, a fruit is supposed to be sweet in taste, and sweetness is its virtue, so don't let the weight-loss industry prejudice you against it. It's through this sweetness that it entices the cells of our body to absorb and assimilate the many phytonutrients it carries. The humble jackfruit has therapeutic nutrients called isoflavones, lignans, and saponins, and all have known anti-cancer properties and an ability to fight 'free radicals' that cause ageing. It's also rich in the micro-mineral copper, which plays a role in thyroid metabolism and thus weight loss. Ha! Now i have your attention!

There's more. It's rich in vitamin B6, so if you have overeaten at dinner, eating this fruit for breakfast will help you beat the gas and acidity that follows. And if you are a protein junkie, then jackfruit seeds roasted or used in curries to be eaten with rice make for the complete amino acid profile. Jackfruit's ability to reverse ageing, lower body fat, keep thyroid healthy and the stomach clear, are not well known, but its sweetness is. So go ahead, savour the fruit for its sweetness; its magical and curative process will be at work silently.

Jackfruit seeds—the true Indian superfood

1. Versatile: Boil them, roast them or cook them in a curry to go with rice.
2. Nutritious:

• Polyphenols that give you ageless skin.
• Zinc and other micro minerals that help boost fertility and hormonal health.
• Fibre, riboflavin and rich vitamin B profile that both reduce and regulate high BP, improve blood sugar control and reduce gut inflammation.
3. Aam aadmi fruit: Easy on the pocket, every part of it is useful, it's zero wastage.

As a team, we often sit together and peel open the jackfruit. We chat about boyfriends, chai, clients. We learn that hard exteriors may be tough to handle but hold the promise of sweetness inside.

Oh btw, monsoon is a great time for jackfruit seeds. Green veggies are off the menu but the seeds ensure a steady supply of vitamins, fibre and minerals.

P.S.: If you follow Shravan, you may also put meat and eggs off the list, and the seeds will ensure a steady supply of amino acids too. They are truly versatile.

Sitaphal

Fruit with epic qualities

When the festive season is upon us—Navratri and Diwali—so will the need to go on a 'diet'. But all you foodies looking for 'accelerated fat metabolism', don't miss out on the sitaphal this season. Goddess Sita has always been worshipped for her calm, commitment and courage, and it is with good reason that the sitaphal has been honoured with her name: literally translated, it means 'Sita's fruit'.

A seasonal fruit, sitaphal is best savoured when the time is right, i.e., when it's in season. But just like mangoes, chickoos and bananas, sitaphal has been deemed a complete no-no if one is on a weight-loss programme. Well, here's some news for all sitaphal critics—this fruit has the goodness of iron, potassium and vitamin B6. All of these are essential nutrients to counter bloating, hair loss and insomnia. Its fibre provides the necessary roughage and B vitamins for your intestines, which otherwise feel dull, overworked and exhausted when on a diet.

Sitaphal, just like apple, papaya or pear, does not contain fat. It just provides our body with natural sugar or fructose, which has a low glycaemic index and results in slow insulin release and accelerated fat-burning. So, sitaphal can actually speed up weight loss. Eat it at the right time: as your first meal, post any physical exercise, or as a whole meal before sunset. In fact, just the sight of a much-loved sitaphal stimulates the secretion of digestive juices, further speeding up digestion and metabolism. Only if you are eating it without any guilt, that is!

Don't shy away from sitaphal—fears and facts

Fear—avoid if diabetic.

Fact—low on glycaemic index (54); not just safe, but foods that are low on the index—55 and below—are recommended for diabetics.

Fear—avoid if fat.

Fact—good source of vitamin B-complex, specially vitamin B6, so even works at reducing bloating.

Fear—avoid if heart patient.
Fact—high on minerals like manganese and vitamin C, has an anti-ageing effect on the heart and circulatory system.
Fear—avoid if you have PCOD.
Fact—good source for iron, fights feelings of tiredness, irritability and improves fertility.

An open letter from khichdi

i am in the news. Like, headline news. How do i feel about it? Nothing different actually. Maybe i am too old to feel excited about a momentary rush, and too laidback to get carried away. But i have a responsibility towards my fellow foods, the neglected, undervalued preparations in this country's kitchens. We don't know when, and if, our turn in the spotlight will come again, so i have to make use of this opportunity. i am going to talk about me, but i represent many. Listen up.

1. Not just food for the sick: Unless of course you count the obese, the diabetics, the heart patients, those with PCOD and thyroid problems, cancer, IBS and many more as sick. That the sick can eat me, even when they don't feel like eating anything else, is my virtue, not a limitation. For centuries though, i have been the preferred dinner option across the country. Easy on the stomach, especially as digestion weakens post sunset, but exciting enough with the ghee, dahi, spices, pickle and papad to cater to all tastes, i hereby lay claim to the best meal for dinner.

2. A balanced meal: The ghee, spices, pickle/papad are not just for excitement, they make me—in language you understand—the most 'balanced meal'. Ghee lowers my glycaemic index, and rice adds a mixture of prebiotics to go with the probiotics like dahi, kadhi, pickle. Now that's balance. The spices add flavour, along with many nutrients, some known to nutrition science, most yet to be discovered, but present in me nevertheless. My power lies in the proportion—little more rice, little less dal, some ghee, a pinch of spices and herbs, a dash of salt—and in its perfectly balanced execution in your kitchen.

3. Future of food: The world is struggling with the triple burden of malnourishment—undernourishment, micronutrient deficiencies and obesity. The scientists say the solution is plant protein. Doctoral theses are being done on the best combinations of pulses, grains and spices which make for perfect meals. My dear countrymen and women, i am the future of food. i am the plant-based protein meal which can help the hungry and overfed. Thank your ancestors for perfecting me over generations, testing and tweaking me in real-life conditions. Now, present me to the world.

4. Simple and diverse: Like the sa of the sargam, you will get the song of your life right if you get me right. An artist will tell you that sa is the foundation, the ever-steady sur, and yet the sa of one raga sounds different from another. Just like the same dal and rice will taste different in a different home, region and community. This is not my failing but my greatest strength. i am food for the rich and the poor, for the devout and the atheist, the toddler

and the ageing. i will blend, but yet stay distinct. i am not just a dish, i am a part of the food system. i am your way of life. i am you.

Kokum

Have you heard of the Konkan? The 'susegad' (relaxed) coast of Maharashtra that extends into Goa? If you have, then you must have heard of kokum. It's a fruit, used as a spice and also to make yummy curries that are eaten with rice. All right, you are not into tourism or cooking, you are into weight loss; so what do we have for you? Here goes. Kokum is great to reduce lipogenesis, i.e. conversion of food to fat. It is rich in many phytonutrients, and this particular fat-loss benefit is brought about by HCA or hydroxycitric acid, which is also found in fancy weight-loss supplements and in ads that pop up every time you open Facebook and urge you to lose thirteen kilos. Wink wink. Jokes apart, HCA is just one of the many ingredients that make kokum revered in south India.

Mentioned in Ayurvedic texts as effective therapy for beating dehydration, flatulence, infections and allergies, it is now also touted for its anti-carcinogenic properties. It has multiple other uses too: for an even skin tone and taking care of enlarged pores. Other than using it as a spice or seasoning, Konkanis eat kokum by converting it into a drink called amrut kokum. Seeped in the right amount of sugar and allowed to settle for some time with cumin and salt, it makes for as delicious a liver cleanser and coolant as you could ask for. Why isn't it popular then, if it's really so great for the skin, intestines and beating the heat? Well, the same can be asked for bel ka sherbet and rhododendron. Blame it on the fact that we don't quite take home-grown food wisdom seriously.

Kokum sherbet

Kokum makes for a beautiful drink to bond over (anxiolytic—inhibits anxiety). It also boosts immunity (Garcinol—fights viral and fungal infections) and is fat-burning (Hydroxy citric acid—natural fat burning agent).

Especially good for:

1. Hormonal disorders and vaginal infections
2. Cholesterol and BP disorders
3. Insulin insensitivity and obesity

Moringa

Beating our own drums

Haldi did it, now it's the turn of the drumstick, called moringa in Tamil and currently the rage across the globe, the new superfood. In our country, however, it has the 'poor man's food' tag. The rich are popping moringa tabs or powder post a run, but don't even know that it's the same drumstick that they remove from their sambar while eating idli.

Indian tribals have used it for centuries as a tree that gives shade in summer, is resilient through the drought and can work as a quick antiseptic or even as a lactation medicine when required. The urban elite, however, scan websites or read fashion magazines instead of looking at nature or natives to learn the art of mental or physical wellbeing. Magazines and websites are hugely inspired by the West, who in turn are looking at tribals of South America, Africa and Asia to fish for the next weight-loss aid. Back it with adequate research, often funded by food and pharma industries, throw in the backing of a celeb and nifty packaging and the 'novel' food is now ready to be sold and consumed. Even in the land it belongs to. But this time as a blood sugar regulator, with antioxidant-rich, anti-ageing compounds and minerals that help prevent bone and joint disorders.

The need of the hour is for big campaigns like #MakeinIndia to showcase native fruits, plants and trees and educate the masses about their benefits. For a diabetic country like ours, the drumstick that goes in sambar, its flowers that blend in an adai or thalipeeth, or the work that the tree does in preserving groundwater, should not go unnoticed. And it is nothing short of ironic if we learn about this from Western media.

Pulses

Top four reasons you must bring pulses back on your plate

1. Pulses are nutrient rich: When we mix pulses and cereals in the right proportion, we create the easy-to-assimilate, high-on-biological-value, plant protein. Whether it's regular food like dal-chawal, khichdi, idli or delicacies like puran poli, dal kachori, etc.

2. Pulses have major health benefits: Pulses are an important source of minerals and help lower blood sugars. They also help prevent adult acne, the type that show up on the chin and upper forehead. They are also the ancient Ayurvedic secret to prevent kidney stones and gall stones.
3. Pulses are generous: By fixing nitrogen back in the soil, they nourish and enrich the soil they grow in and, in turn, sustain the entire ecosystem of the region—flowers, fruits, bees, etc. This also ensures chemical fertilisers are not needed.
4. Pulses are cool: If you like hashtagging what you eat, all the latest trends—#vegan #dairyfree #glutenfree #crueltyfree—apply to pulses.

India had more than 65,000 varieties of pulses, we barely eat six now. Bring back at least twelve to fifteen pulses in your life and it will not only increase the diversity and strength of your gut bacteria, but also support local farmers and improve global ecology. It's a win-win.

P.S.: The Canada food guide 2019 (considered amongst the best in the world for nutrition advice) called it both a vegetable and a protein for its amino acid profile, vitamin B and fibre.

Sweet Potato

The magic of sweet potato

Anna is the sarvottam aushadha; food is the best medicine, say the scriptures. The one that is grown in your soil, fresh in the season and eaten with gratitude, says both our culture and common sense.

Ratala, ratalu, shakarkandi, sweet potato is here, but where are you?

- The fibrous vegetable is safe for everyone to eat, the ones battling obesity, PCOD, diabetes especially.
- Makes for a great snack and allows for quick recovery from training.
- The vitamin A will fight all infections, the anthocynins will keep your skin supple, the minerals and vitamin B profile will keep the bloating, acidity and constipation away.
- Basically, if you have drunk too much, slept too little and partied too hard, this is what you should be eating.

Jaggery

The many wonders of jaggery

Winter brings not just the chills but also the harvest of sugarcane. This is also why from Tulsi puja (end of Diwali) till almost Holi, jaggery occupies the position of prasad (an honour reserved for the harvest of the season and gratitude for the farmer).

Cultural aspect aside, jaggery is celebrated across regions. In Uttar Pradesh, families and neighbours get together while the jaggery is being prepared and roll it into medium-sized balls, like laddoos. This then becomes an 11 a.m. snack when farmers take a break and it's to be enjoyed with a glass of water. In Maharashtra, in summer, when you have a guest over or kids are back after playing for a long time, it's a practice to first bite into jaggery and then have water.

While jaggery is known for its many benefits, i wonder if the summer practice in Maharashtra and farming practice in UP indicate the thermal-regulatory properties of jaggery. And in that case, it would be a good meal to have if you are breaking into a sweat over nothing.

But stories apart, have the jaggery for it can:

- improve your skin.
- prevent dandruff and hair fall.
- and give relief from bloating and constipation.

Bhakri or roti with jaggery, and ghee or peanuts with jaggery are the most non-fussy combos.

But if you are in a mood for something more sophisticated, try this variant from UP. It's fresh jaggery mixed with soonth (dry ginger powder), til and peanuts. You cut it in shapes of your choice and if you store it in an airtight container, it has a long shelf life.

And if you wake up sloppy and hungover on 1st January, have one. How's that for a free recommendation for a hangover?

Laddoos

The annual breastfeeding week (August 1–7) advocates the benefits of breast milk to the baby and the mother. The process of lactation is natural, of course, but there are a few things that can either enhance or come in its way.

Nutrition schools teach you that a lactating mother needs at least 500 Kcal more than normal. This is to let the mother recover from the physiological stress of delivery and the sleepless nights that come with having a baby. It also allows for a better return to hormonal balance and pre-pregnancy weight and the extra energy that is required to produce milk.

In India, however, you don't pop pills, shakes or simply eat more to achieve this state of energy balance. You work your way through it by mixing nutrients in the most delicious concoctions. Native cultures understand that science must be practical if it has to sustain real life, or else it's lost in papers and labs.

Two ways in which dadi and nani rose to the occasion are:

Gond laddoo: Made from a natural gum and mixed with nuts, it strengthens the spine and makes up for the loss of bone density during pregnancy.

Aliv laddoo: Garden cress seed, a rich source of iron, mixed with coconut and coconut water. Makes up for blood loss during and post pregnancy. The coconut water literally squeezes all the bloating out of you. (Give it to your teenage daughter too—it beats pimples and PMS.)

Laddoos are not just tasty but can be eaten at any time, including the middle of the night without waking up the household. It's a guilt-free, disease-free way of beating midnight blues, and unlike chocolate and ice cream, it doesn't show up on your waistline.

Aliv

Aliv, the secret beauty pill

Taken in the form of a laddoo, ideally, along with coconut, jaggery and ghee. Rolled with bare hands, with love in your heart and a smile on your lips.

1. MUST for every pre-pubescent boy and girl so that they don't fall short on iron and make a smooth transition to puberty with robust Hb levels.
2. MUST for every teenager: the folate will ensure that even when you have a breakup, you don't have break-outs.
3. MUST for every couple who are planning to make babies. It's the best-kept fertility secret.
4. MUST for everyone at peri and post menopause, as the sulforaphane helps prevent and clear pigmentation on the skin.

P.S.: A fav snack on my morning flights. Prevents acidity, bloating and other travel headaches.

FAQs on aliv

Q. Who can have aliv?

Everyone, especially lactating women, children reaching puberty, adults facing hair loss, patchy skin, alopecia, etc. It also helps in de-stressing. Rich in folic acid, iron, vitamin E and vitamin A, so, very good for immunity too.

Q. How to have aliv?

Always with essential fat. For example, aliv laddoo made of ghee, coconut, jaggery as a mid-meal snack, or soaked aliv seeds (a small pinch) with milk at bedtime.

Q. How much aliv to have?
Just a pinch of soaked aliv seeds in milk or in time-tested proportions in the laddoo, kheer, etc. Don't overdo it.

RECIPE FOR ALIV LADDOO

Ingredients:

Aliv seeds, 1 katori
1 big coconut, grated
Jaggery, 2½ katori (can vary as per sweetness of gur)
Ghee, 2 teaspoons
Jaiphal powder

Steps:

- Soak the aliv for one hour in coconut water.
- Mix the grated coconut and gur in the soaked aliv.
- After half an hour, cook the mixture in a kadhai with the ghee.
- Continue heating till mixture gets cooked properly.
- Allow to cool, add jaiphal powder and roll into laddoos.
- If kept in a refrigerator, it will stay good for ten days. If kept outside, for three days.

Til/Sesame

- Reduces inflammation.
- Low glycaemic index, improves insulin sensitivity.
- Mineral-rich, improves fertility.
- Calcium-rich, great for bones and thyroid health.

• Has essential fatty acids that improve cardio-vascular health.
• Has phytonutrients that prevent hair fall and dandruff.

Winter food that has weathered the storm of many diet fads—the West calls it sesame and the food of the future.

TIL, CHOTE SIZE MEIN BADA RECHARGE

Til has the fibre and minerals that nourish both the body and the brain. While it allows the thinking parts of the brain to be better connected, it provides the body with more suppleness and prevents pigmentation of the skin. In a way, it's amongst the most underrated anti-ageing food produce.

When i was in Kuwait for a private talk, i was given their version of til wadi, offered and eaten as a dessert or with Arabic coffee or simply as a mid-meal snack. It's amazing that while India has a full-fledged festival dedicated to it, Sankranti, every native culture has its own version of this tiny little seed.

And since we are all products of what we eat, the cultural and social similarities between us and the Arab world are quite strong. Essentially, it means that we are all the same from within, but like the til, based on the region we come from, we appear in different forms, sizes and shapes. It's the external diversity that we must celebrate and hold the internal sameness close to our hearts.

Mango curry

Kairi curry or mango curry served on hot rice with ghee will melt in your mouth. But the goodness doesn't just stop there, it gives a boost to your skin, helps liver function and even prevents constipation.

The key though is to chew slowly, relish every bite and to feel grateful for the presence of mango in your life. And also for the presence of our foremothers who used the mango at every stage—raw, ripe, overripe—and turned it into delicacies that people of all age groups can enjoy.

In effect, they helped optimise the nutrients from this seasonal produce, prevented wastage and left a good taste in our mouths for generations to come.

The mango is not a king for nothing. It was crowned by the women of India, Africa and other parts of Asia because of its versatility, good looks and vast resource of nutrients.

Dig in folks, for the goodness has withstood every test.

P.S.: Recipe shared by Shravani Sawant on my Insta page:

In Karwar we call it sasav. A paste of sankeshwari mirchi, coriander seeds, green chillies, freshly grated coconut and couple of garlic cloves are ground in a stone grinder (you can also grind it in a mixer.) And for the tadka we can use kachi ghani coconut oil, splatter some mustard seeds, curry leaves, a pinch of hing and add the paste. Add the small tropical mangoes, also known as bitka amba or aam at some places, which are half ripened so that you get a tangy sweet, sour and hot mango curry or sasav.

Ber

Benefits of eating ber:

- Strengthens the immune system (great for those who fall sick frequently).
- Rich in vitamin C (richer than oranges), lethal for dandruff and the secret behind glowing skin.
- Magic cure for constipation.

Kaddu

Coughing this season, catching a cold or feeling a bit under the weather?

Here is the answer to all your troubles—kaddu, bhopla, pumpkin my munchkins.

The richest source of vitamin A, carotenes, xanthin and zeaxanthin, the pumpkin will help fight infections, boost your immunity and speed up recovery.

The vitamins B and the B6 especially will help cut down bloating and ease PMS pain. The folate will help improve iron assimilation, improve Hb levels and leave you feeling fresh and free of acne and dandruff this season.

The pumpkin can turn into anything you fancy:

Pooris, that are popular with kids.

Sabzi, curry, sambar, popular with adults.

Halwa, that's popular with everyone.

Alright then, what's stopping you?

In a side note, do note that our English language science textbooks fail to mention kaddu as the richest source of vitamin A, and we are stuck with carrots in our heads because it made its way to the syllabus.

The next time you think carrots for A, spinach for Fe and oranges for C, ask yourself if it's because it's true or because it was in your textbook?

Sabudana

Everywhere i go (or used to go before Covid-19), women tell me that now that they have turned forty they want to do something for themselves.

Toh, this is what i think you should do. Make sabudana wada for yourself. If this is not an act of liberation, courage and finally coming of age, i don't know what is.

And while you are at it, know that when they told you that sabudana is all empty calories, they lied. Sabudana, with jeera, kadi patta, mirchi, namak, peanut powder and coconut chutney, is the stuff that happiness is made of. Which is why traditionally it also qualifies as a fasting food. It promotes hormonal balance in women.

Especially helpful in case of: 1. Hot flushes 2. Excessive bleeding that goes on for days together 3. High testosterone levels.

Happy eating, happy rediscovering the many glories of Indian food.

P.S.: In the future, when you hear about casava as a superfood, think of this post.

P.P.S.: NY Times has already carried an article on subudana khichdi.

Onions

Rich in biotin, B6 and B1, onions are just what nature ordered for silky hair and strong nails.

The polyphenols are known to prevent ageing and reduce oxidative stress, thus protecting you from high blood sugar and even heart diseases.

Onions enable the liver to metabolise fat better and should be on your plate if you are fighting a fatty liver. It also helps regulate cholesterol levels.

Onions, especially the white ones, are a traditional medicine to reduce heat in the body, and overcome heat stroke and fatigue in the harsh summer.

For best results, hold it in one hand, squash it with the other and eat it with your bhakri and chutney.

Misal

Some people spend a lifetime looking for a guru or grace or simply a good turn of destiny, but it never seems to come their way.

And mostly the reason for that is that they are never looking for what is already on their plate. Take the case of misal, a mixture of sprouts, cooked well with a delicious mix of spices, garnished with farsan, dhaniya, tomato, kanda. Bole toh life mein aur kya chahiye, bhidu? Aur mang ne pe, iss ke saath pav ya dahi bhi mil sakta hai.

The key then is to keep your senses sharp, heart open and hands clean so that when grace or guru or destiny arrives in the form of misal, you are not caught napping, counting calories or in search of avocado and millet risotto or whatever. That when misal arrives you see it as the brilliance of the collective wisdom of our grandmoms. That you don't miss its super amino acid or micronutrient profile just because it's dressed unlike how superfoods are supposed to.

After all, it would be silly to not recognise regional and traditional dishes for the health and happiness they bring to all who will bite into them.

When was the last time you relished a real good misal? When was the last time you recognised that grace, guru or even God is already present in the fleeting moments of life? When was the last time that you lived your life with an open heart?

Bel

The bel sherbet

You won't find billboard ads that declare its purity. They won't serve you this at your first class seat as it's so nutrient-rich that it will perish in the logistical chain. It's so exotic and seasonal that the Insta generation hasn't even learnt that it's pout- and pose-worthy.

But all this means nothing for the bel or the wood apple or Japanese bitter orange. It has seen it all, from the time of the Vedas and the Mahabharata, and it is confident that the new India will see, sooner rather than later, that content is invaluable and packaging is rubbish. That richness or coolness comes from adopting the local and native and not from copying a trend. More importantly, the bel knows that the wise men and women of north India still have its sherbet every morning to beat the heat. The bel knows that it's future-proof, that with climate change, it's therapeutic value will be yearned by all.

Here are some things you should know:

- Offers instant relief from constipation and bloating.
- Rich in antioxidants; helps regulate blood sugar and reduces risks and complications that arise out of diabetes.
- Rich in carotene; protects the heart, nerves and eyes.
- Prevents hair fall, dandruff and reduces pigmentation of the skin.
- Great to taste, good for the local economy and preserves the ecology.

Look it up and drink up its goodness. Life doesn't get better than this.

Raisins

The power of black raisins

Yeh chota bomb, kare bade kaam.

- Black raisins—the traditional medicine for frizzy hair, painful periods and excessive bleeding.
- Also works wonders for constipation, bloating and mood swings.
- Best enjoyed when soaked overnight and placed between a mamra badam, soaked overnight and peeled.

This is how i start my day, what about you?

Nimbu

The superfood test

1. Versatility: can you use this one thing to make multiple things?
Yes—sherbet, achaar, garnishing.
2. Does it have medicinal/therapeutic properties?
Yes—from eye health to dandruff, the nimbu can resolve it all. Which is also why nimbu mirchi can rid you from buri nazar.
But ya, if you have the problem of an oily scalp that goes with dry hair that has split ends, then bathe with hot water in which you have squeezed nimbu and watch the magic in just three weeks.
3. Art: is the food referenced in art? Does it have a kahawat? A song? A motif that appears on sarees? A toran that hangs on doors?
Well, nimbu has songs rich in folklore. The most popular being Madhuri Dixit's *Woh kharbuja laya joh nimbu mangaye*.

So by the powers vested in me (by myself), i declare nimbu a superfood. Do you concur? What's your fav thing about nimbu?

Dahi

The test of good, homemade dahi is that the spoon resting on top of it shouldn't sink.

Because dahi has the force to uplift more than just your spirits. It uplifts your ability to stay steady in a world of constant change, it protects gut integrity and gut bacteria diversity. Need more reasons to dig in?

P.S.: Test not applicable for packaged dahi.

Aloo paratha

Was my post-workout meal today. Typically, i stick to sevaiya upma or poha, but today was special. There was a chill in the air, time on hand and a chuha in the stomach.

Routinely people write to me—i have been put on a diet and my rotis have been stopped, can't live like this forever, what should i do?

Very simply, listen to yourself, your heritage and lineage, over anybody else. And follow the basics:

- Buy gehu, not atta.
- Peeso it in the neighbourhood chakki.
- Store it in a nice steel dabba.
- And every time you take the atta out, use clean hands and a dry spoon.

Simple enough?

Then roll it into a dough the usual way with the tel (or ghee), namak, water, and make just enough to last you for that one meal or at the most for that one day. The fresher, the better.

Winters are also the time for parathas—aloo, mooli, kulith ka parathas. They taste great with achaar and chutneys, keep your body strong and stomach light.

Use the iron tava and it's best eaten piping hot.

Oats vs traditional breakfasts

The easy answer to: Should i replace my traditional breakfast with oats?

No.

Why?

Not tasty.

Need more?

Don't blend with regional cuisine and cooking methods. Don't grow in the soil close to you or if they are grown don't support the ecological diversity. Not in sync with the climate. Available in packaged form only. Nutrient profile on paper not the same as what gets assimilated inside the body. Excess fibre comes in the way of nutrient absorption.

But what about convenience?

Poha, upma, idli, dalia, etc., are equally, if not more, convenient and quick to prepare.

P.S.: The nutrition profile that oats sell themselves on already exists in our traditional breakfast options, which are much tastier too. Oats, in fact, tried to become more like our traditional foods with the addition of herbs and spices, and there are plenty of masala versions in the market now.

Neem and the bitter truth about the superfoods of India

The neem and every part of the tree has been celebrated for its anti-inflammatory, anti-allergic and analgesic properties since time immemorial in India. It's been a part of our folklore, food and festivals. Some regions, like Hyderabad, make a special drink from the neem flowers that blossom during this season and Bengal turns the tender leaves into a speciality sabzi to be enjoyed with aamras and poori. Both help the body stay in tune with the change in season, and not get bloated, acidic or dehydrated in response to the heat.

Now, as we turn our back on traditions, we are turning into a population that chews raw salads for lunch and pops a neem tablet for health. The same is valid for haldi tablets or consuming huge amounts of flaxseed/jeera/cinnamon with water. Or for that matter, starting the day with coconut oil or adding ghee to coffee. Basically, trying to maximise the intake of a particular food/nutrient for the perceived benefit of weight loss, detox or what not.

The truth, though, is that health doesn't lie in isolated compounds of our native produce but in its link to our food combinations and cuisines.

The food industry teaches us to be greedy. Time-tested food traditions teach us to be in tune with nature and enjoy what's on our plate. The choice is simple.

Turmeric

An open letter from haldi

Hey you! Yes, you, checking out the curcumin pill in the supermarket aisle. That's not how i am pronounced. But then this is also not where i am found. Once upon a time, i enjoyed a rather enviable place in the kitchen, sorry, hearts of people. If you had a cut, i was there to heal it. If you were getting married, i was a part of the festivities. If you couldn't sleep, i was there to soothe you. Your dals, sabzis, even poojas were incomplete without me.

Now the woke have woken up to my glories and i am being industrialised as a commodity that removes inflammation, infection and boosts immunity. In the Western world, i can now be found as part of breakfast cereals and lattes and am shot up in the morning with a glass of water. i have also been turned into gels, pills and pumps.

But what breaks my heart is the way people i consider mine, the ones i soothed, celebrated and healed, treat me. They don't call me by my name now but i am referred to as a product. The pandemic has meant the launch of turmeric lattes in India. India? i am living my nightmare, really. We have lost so much pride, and more importantly, common sense, that we are now copying the people who copied us. And instead of figuring that we are losing perspective, we are patting our backs saying 'hum toh pehle se hi karte the'.

Where's your accountability for God's sake? i didn't flinch when you stopped using me in sabzis as you replaced them with a salad. When you traded haldi milk for chamomile tea, i didn't sit in a corner and cry. When you used creams instead of me on your skin, i didn't complain. You know why? Not because i lacked confidence to speak up but because i was compassionate and understanding of the fact that this is how colonised countries behave. They look down upon their own, they trade them for poorer but 'master'-approved stuff—be it produce or people.

i have been around for thousands of years and i have seen a lot; a decade or two of being neglected or underutilised didn't faze me. Not just because i am extremely powerful and ancient but also because i knew you would come around. Come around to realising that you have been neglecting priceless wisdom just because it's transmitted as an oral tradition, in a native language and by women. And that you would also realise that health is built on a foundation of culture, crop-cycle and climate and it is furthered by gender equality, native cuisines and languages. Food traditions, when used to their full potential, not only lead to thriving health but also boost local economy and protect ecology. This pandemic was your chance to relearn that.

Instead, you appropriated me, reduced me to just one of my molecules, branded and packaged me and acted like you gifted me to the world. You made me into who i am not. This gel, this shot, this pill and this pandemic is on you.

—Haldi

RUJUTA SAYS...

Knowing how to roll an aliv laddoo in your hands is cooler than swirling a 'vintage' wine in your mouth!

Moramba, chundo and achaar—you are blessed if you still practice the art of making one of these anti-ageing secrets that your grandma left behind.

When you are served with love and you eat with gratitude, you should count your blessings and not carbs, fat and protein. Much less calories. :-)

Sweet potato during the Navratra ensures that women (men too) get their dose of vitamin B and magnesium and prevents aches and pains during the winter that follows.

Kesar (saffron) with 150+ volatile aromatic oils can lift you out of depression and give your skin that taut, well hydrated look. Kewah anyone?

Not all scientists work in labs, speak in English and write in journals. Some work on farms and put food on your plate.

2D. FORGOTTEN SUPERFOODS

Gopa poori

Liberating, uplifting and empowering. That's exactly what the Indian food culture means to me. This poori is just one of the many dry nashta delicacies that women in Indian kitchens designed, perfected and practised. It meant that the whole household had access to nutritious mid-meals that could be enjoyed over chai and charcha. It could also be offered to anyone who dropped by to your home. Or it even worked as a token of love that you carried as a guest to someone else's home.

India's dry nashta tradition—basically, non-perishables cooked as savouries, sweets, etc.—is a testimony to the adventure, versatility and creativity of Indian women and their kitchens. The trend of eating only two meals a day and claiming it to be a cultural practice is just another testament of how women's contributions to health and wellbeing are ignored and rubbished routinely by the weight-loss industry and its influencers.

This one in particular is special, it's made especially during mango season and gopa poori and aamras are a super speciality of Saurashtra in Gujarat.

Dawa chi chutney

This is chutney made from harabara (chickpea) leaves that are plucked early in the morning when the dew settles on them.

These are now called as forgotten foods and to bring them back in focus, the UNFAO had declared 2016 as the year of pulses. Pulses don't just fix the nitrogen back into our soils naturally but also provide critical amino acids to the body. Their leaves are a good source of minerals. But all that jazz aside, i loved the taste of the morning dew chutney; never before had i eaten anything more exotic, crunchier and flavourful.

Patoli

Sometimes i wonder if we, as people, as a culture and country, are poor at marketing our skills and wisdom. i mean, people go to Paris to become pastry chefs and learn packaging and they find a steady clientele and money by putting together Diwali gifts, etc. In the meanwhile, handcrafted laddoos, barfis, halwas and sheeras not only disappear from the goodie bag but also from the sweet shop shelves and even our kitchens.

But then, i remind myself that food cultures are interwoven in our DNA. Our food traditions are not for recipe books, they are coded in our genes. Our food rituals are not mastered with certifications but are alive for generations through stories, memories and generosity of sharing.

A beautiful patoli came to me in a steel dabba that smelled of love. The coconut, jaggery and chana dal mixture melted in my mouth with the sweetness of its coastal origins. The haldi leaves left an imprint on the rice flour covering and sparkled with the intelligence of eating the harvest of the season.

Cupcakes with their food colouring and fancy moulds may be more Instagrammable, but the naturally tainted delicacies with leaves, spices and love will outlive us and every trend.

Because wisdom is unseen, steady and sweet. You may not be aware of it, but it remains aware of you. And when you are ready, it will come to you and melt in your mouth.

Amboli—the original instant (but healthy) breakfast

Diet trends are temporary, breakfast is permanent.

Amongst the countless speciality food items in our country, a large majority are for breakfast. There are options for every possible situation—a big celebration, a festival, an upvaas, limited time to cook, and many more.

One such time-tested, heritage breakfast preparation is amboli. It's a mixture of rice, pulses, herbs and spices, and once prepared can be cooked into a delicious meal in less than five minutes.

What is the special breakfast preparation of your region which is similar to amboli? Let me know.

And remember—don't skip breakfast. Have a hot, homemade breakfast every day.

RECIPE FOR AMBOLI

Step 1: Making amboli flour

Ingredients:

Rice (preferably patni variety), 5 katori
Chana dal, 1 katori
Udal dal, 1 katori
Coriander seeds, ⅓ katori
Methi seeds, 2 teaspoons

- Grind all the above together.
- Keep in an airtight container (glass bottle).

Step 2: Making amboli

- Add water and a little chaas/curd to the flour, and keep aside for one hour.
- Add chilli powder, salt, haldi and garlic (crushed).
- Now heat an iron/cast iron tawa, add a little oil and spread it over the tawa.
- Now spread one big spoon of the above mixture on the tawa and cover with the lid.
- Heat on a low flame.
- After one side is done, turn it over and heat for another two minutes.
- Now remove from the tawa and eat with ghee and mirchi pickle.

Konfal

Don't ask me what it's called in English, listen to what i am telling you and eat veggies that have no name in English. Speak about food in your local, regional language. One that connects you with your culture, cuisine, crop cycle and climate.

Traditionally, the arrival of monsoon meant eating less green, leafy vegetables and more creeper vegetables like doodhi and root vegetables (and tubers like konfal). Monsoon also signalled the arrival of chaturmas (four months), a period of many festivals and upavas or fasts (not to be confused with the trend of fasting where the focus is to go long hours without food in the name of cleanse or weight loss).

These fasts and what to eat during them are a cultural practice that has stood the test of time and is rooted in common sense. They introduced diversity in our diets in the form of tubers, pulses and smaller millets. The tubers were especially important as the fasts asked you to eat a variety of those. Nutrition science now recognises them as good sources of prebiotic (food for healthy and diverse gut bacteria), isoflavones (that allow for hormonal wellbeing) and a variety of vitamins and minerals that improve blood sugar response.

Unfortunately, a lot of our vegetables, tubers especially, are losing out as we now speak of food mostly in English. So, the broccoli, kale, etc. thrive, while the native species die. This monsoon, bring back the tubers that are a part of your region and culture.

Kusum—the beauty fruit

Check out this micro berry, kusum, as the tribals call it in Sonave. It's a wild, uncultivated fruit that grows in the forests of Maharashtra, all over India and Southeast Asia in fact.

The girls will eat it for the sweet-sour, playful taste and turn the seeds into earrings. It's the fruit for the beautiful, they will tell you. And if you check its therapeutic properties, its linked to preventing hair loss and acne that is caused by androgens. Interesting, isn't it?

When you go for a trek in the Sahyadri this monsoon, look for this beauty.

Balam kakdi

So i may or may not ever find my balam but i am happy to announce to the world that i have found my balam kakdi, at lunch in Indore.

Balam kakdi—first of all, i didn't even know that you exist but then it was truly love at first sight. With one bite, i was transformed, taken to a world of sweetness, joy and hydration. (It's like a mix of kakdi, melon and papaya.)

How seamlessly and sweetly you, a native of Indore, must have lowered core body temperatures of the Indoris in the sweltering October heat. So generous, so kind, i thought to myself. School kids, athletes and BP patients who struggle with bloating and headaches ought to discover you.

Madaula

Meet this wild child, madaula. An uncultivated and wild flower that blooms all over in the Himalaya in the spring season.

The Himachali people relish it as a sabzi or pakoda. It blooms with sunshine, closes without it.

It's these native species that are the unsung heroes of our diet diversity, health and ecology.

Kong—a forgotten millet, especially healthy for menopausal women

You probably haven't heard of it. At least i hadn't until a client gifted it to me last month, fresh from his farm. Not too many of us in Gujarat grow this now, he said. 'Ab iska bhaav nahi nikalta, demand is low, only a few families still eat it.'

Kong, a millet, looks and tastes like a cousin of vari, samo or jhangora. It's eaten as an alternative to rice during fasts, especially during festivals like Navratri. You can make it like khichdi or a Gujarati speciality called khais, where it is cooked with buttermilk.

Millets are important for everyone because of their vitamin B, fibre and mineral profile. It helps children with their immunity, older adults with bone density and even works as a cardio protective agent.

But in peri-menopausal and menopausal women, it is most useful. It has:

- Phenolics that protect the skin from discolouration and ageing.
- Lignans that protect from hormone-based cancers.
- Vitamins B6 and B1 can prevent migraines, bloating and inflammation.

Moving away from traditional foods reduces farming of traditional foods, which in turn has an adverse effect on soil health and ecology, putting not just our health but our entire future at risk.

Jaam—keep calm and eat jaam

They say that there are two sides to every coin. So while the coronavirus may slow you down and force you to stay indoors, don't let it shut the doors on curiosity and cheerfulness.

In spring time, if you look outside, you will see a beauty in bloom. It's the hyperlocal fruit of this season—jaam or rose apple as some people call it. It will turn into a tasty, crunchy, pinkish fruit that is so powerful in its nutrients that it will ensure that you will stay in the pink of health, now and forever.

It's time to reinforce that longevity, immunity and cohesion in society is born out of sharing all that is local, seasonal and traditional.

Stronger together, safer together, smarter together.

Suran

Every shoulder and hip is unique and so is suran. The good old vegetable that has been cultivated since forever in Asia, Africa and Latin America is fast losing its glam to the asparagus and broccolis of the world. So here's a quick reminder from the soil about why you should eat the good old suran.

1. You are a little boy/girl and you are shooting up? Well, you need the suran to continue giving you the hormonal boost to get taller, leaner and stronger.

2. You are not old but have started looking older than your age—skin sags, pigments and feels rough? Suran again, with its isoflavones, will give your skin a taut, smooth and soft appearance.
3. You just are a little biggish on the stomach sometimes because your digestion is unpredictable or you have full-blown IBS? Suran again, to rebuild your digestive processes and even to provide good food to your gut-friendly bacteria.
4. Cancer, heart diseases, obesity or diabetes? Suran has the right mix of fibre, minerals, vitamins and phytonutrients to help you tide over your condition.

Probably India's most original mock meat, this was often used in meat-eating families on days they chose to go without meat (aaj mera somvaar, mangalvaar variety). Celebrated in our region as a 'fast food' too, which allows you access to all nutrients without eating much, like during Shravan, Navratri, etc. Can turn into a sabzi, shallow-fried like chips with rice atta or rava—a quick snack for the kid when they get home from school or sports or for the granddad when he comes back from his hospital visit.

Like the shoulder and the hip, the suran has multiple applications too. Eat it yet?

P.S.: Hey! Don't forget to add kokum or amsul when cooking it.

Mulberry

The developed world has a unique problem—it's expensive to eat healthy and almost impossible to source locally grown, fresh food without paying through your nose. Countries like India don't have that kind of a problem. Rich food is still inexpensive, free almost, and easily accessible to all of us. What is misplaced though is our idea of healthy and even richness.

The shehtooth, tooth or toti, the many names that it goes by, is abundantly available everywhere in our part of the world. All we need now is the education and awareness that this fruit is not just super healthy but bloody priceless. Here's why:

1. If you are old and your eye sight is weak—carotenes and zeaxanthin that help keep the retina healthy.
2. You are just a kid and fall sick every change of season—this is the best vitamin shot that you can take that will keep you free from flu and congestion this season.
3. You are just wanting to lose weight but keep feeling bloated—improves digestion and has anti-inflammatory properties which will actually reduce the swelling and help you feel lighter.
4. You are in love—stand under the tree, pluck its fruit and chew on it slowly; your lips will get coloured and the anti-ageing properties of this fruit will make everything seem brighter and happier, even your dushman.
5. You just want a disease-free life—from cancer to diabetes, cholesterol to BP, this fruit will regulate and protect you against all diseases. It has the polyphenols, anthocyanins, fibre to keep every disease, even depression at bay.

Ramphal

The magic of ramphal

Ramphal goes by many other names—bullock's heart or Annona reticulata, but no matter the name, this fruit is just so good to taste and has so many medicinal and therapeutic benefits (like all native, forgotten fruits).

• Pre-diabetic or diabetic and still wondering which is the best fruit for you? This is the one, with its minerals and blood glucose-lowering properties, just what the doctor ordered (except that he didn't—local fruits have no sponsors, so no awareness). Also has anti-cancer properties.

• Frizzy hair, acne marks and weak joints? Allow the ramphal and its nutrients, especially its free radical fighting vitamin C, to help you.

• Poor immune system and fall sick with every weather change? Ramphal again. Its vitamin A will not just boost immunity but its B vitamins will help cut down the inflammation too.

• If you are above thirty and just popped a pimple, then welcome to adult acne and this is the timeless fruit with its buttery inside that will bring your glow back.

Look for ramphal in the old vegetable and fruit markets and bring these native beauties back on your plate.

Tondli

The tiny cylindrical tondli is a storehouse of vitamins B1 and B2 and minerals like iron. The next time you suffer from fatigue and bloating during PMS, or just need something that kick-starts your metabolism, reach out for this vegetable.

Bharali tondli—a preparation with peanuts, coconut and finely calibrated spices—is my favourite. So is tondli bhat. Or i just steam some tondli with salt and have it as a mid-meal snack. What's your favourite?

Cheekh/colostrum

The benefits of the forgotten superfood cheekh, bari or colostrum are immeasurable and the taste is divine. But alas, the kharvas, a delicacy made from colostrum, is fast fading from our kitchen, recipe books and memories. Made from the first milk of a cow, this is diluted with regular milk and cooked patiently and skilfully into pure gold.

- It works as both a pre- and pro-biotic, ensures that your gut bacterial diversity sustains itself and thrives.
- It protects children from falling sick often, and therefore the onslaught of antibiotics. It prevents and eases IBS trouble and reduces dependence on antacids.
- It improves iron assimilation and prevents acne, alopecia and dull skin.

RECIPE FOR KHARVAS

Ingredients:

Cheekh, 1 katori (first day after delivery of cow/ buffalo)
Milk, 1.5 to 2 katoris
Sugar, ½ katori
Kesar or nutmeg or cardamom powder, or a mixture of all three, depending on the individual choice.
Instead of sugar, jaggery can also be used.

Steps:

- Mix well.
- Pressure cook (three whistles) and cut into pieces.

Buckwheat

Trekking in the remote Himalayas may seem like no more than an adventure activity that burns tons of calories, but for me, it's a journey that drives home the philosophy of simplicity or 'eat local, think global'. i just got back from Jolingkong, at the base of Adi-Kailash mountain in Kumaon, right on the Indo-Tibetan border, where i stayed in the wood-and-stone village of Kuti for a couple of nights, mainly to acclimatise to the high altitude. It is here that i tasted the same rotis that sage Vyas, who authored the Mahabharata and lent the valley his name, ate every single day, centuries ago. Made out of kuttu ka atta (buckwheat flour), they were not only rich in calcium, magnesium, iron, fibre, essential fatty acids and vitamin B, but were also flavourful. i ate them with curd that had a tadka of jeera and local greens similar to mustard leaves. It is pretty much this food which nourished the sage, who is revered for his understanding of not just the Vedas, but warfare, geography, ethics and politics.

Little wonder then that men with real insights have the wisdom to eat simple, local food. Kuttu ka atta has all the nutrients to keep the brain sharp, joints lubricated and skin protected from dryness and sun damage. Also, the phytonutrients in kuttu strengthen arteries and lower blood pressure, thus aiding acclimatisation. There's a reason why local food is better than its exotic avatar: it helps you cope with local environmental challenges, be it altitude, heat, cold or humidity. So take a leaf out of rishi Vyas's book and go back to eating local.

Lotus seeds

It felt surreal walking by a Dal Lake awash with lotus blooms and shikaras (made unforgettable by the late Shammi Kapoor). In the middle of my reverie, a vendor waves a green bunch in my face. 'Lotus seed, just Rs 20, try,' he says, pulling out a tiny yellowish seed from the fibrous stem. 'Super! i'll buy it,' i promptly comply. My interest in the lotus seed is varied—it is fresh, seasonal, inexpensive (only Rs 20 for a bunch of four), yummy, and most importantly, brilliant as an anti-ageing agent.

Lotus seeds are rich in vital nutrients and come armed with a special enzyme that actually repairs damaged proteins. This means it helps you look younger. In Kashmir, the lotus seed is eaten both 'because it grows here' and also for its liver-cleansing, kidney-flushing, heart-strengthening properties. It is a goldmine in the offing, which only needs good packaging, positioning and an entrepreneur to fashion it into a flourishing industry. Maybe i can do it, i think. But then, it's easy to dream amidst nature. i am, after all, a middle-class Maharashtrian with zero enterprise!

So, i am writing about it—in the hope that the Kashmir government or a cooperative group actually starts selling it to the rest of the country. It's amazing how 'imported' oils, seeds, leaves and roots get our instant respect, while desi wisdom is casually dismissed. Ayurveda and yoga hold the pamposh, or the lotus, in high esteem, not just for its beauty and as a symbol of purity, but for its therapeutic properties too. When your liver and kidneys are clean and your heart strong, it's easier to enjoy your wealth. That's why Goddess Lakshmi has a lotus seat.

Dates

The rains wash away all that is old and bring not just fresh beginnings but also fresh dates. Celebrated since time immemorial as boosters of fertility, immunity and sensitivity, these little beings are worth their weight in gold.

Fibre: the perfect mix of the soluble and insoluble, it will keep constipation, bloating and irritability away.

Minerals: calcium and magnesium that let you sport a toned look, help cut down the flab and ensure that you stay away from midnight cramps.
Vitamin rich: will prevent skin damage, repair frizzy hair and the B6 will keep your mood in a great place.

How much is too much?

On a trip to Jordan, i learnt the golden Arabic rule—eat the second date only if you can eat the third one. So in that land, it's not allowed to stop at two, you have to eat the third or the fifth or the seventh. So if you feel that you can eat two but not three, then Arab culture says, stop at one. Much like the mitahar concept in the *Hatha Yoga Pradipika*—develop the sensitivity to leave the stomach half empty/half full and share the bounty with the world.

Karonda

Karvanda or karonda is the local coastal berry that you find only in the monsoon. It provides the perfect detox post binge-eating, and it's a balm for the broken heart and stabiliser of blood sugar too. Folk medicine considers it to be a boon for fertility and even calls it 'dongrachi maina' or the bird of the mountains :-). Have you eaten one yet or are you waiting for the West to go gaga over it?

Butta

Maka/makai/butta has the vitamin B and folic acid required to give you good hair and prevent greying, the fibre to rid you of constipation and the taste to soothe and regulate your blood glucose levels. Have it roasted or boiled, turn them into pattice or rotis and enjoy them in full glory. American corn, popcorn and the like—please excuse me, i am not talking about you. i am talking about my beautiful pearly white ones; local rules!

Paan

We learn in school that the first step of digestion is in our mouth. When the tongue feels stimulated by the taste of food, it sends a signal to the brain to secrete the right digestive juices and enzymes. This process is essential for assimilation of nutrients and elimination of waste. So you 'by-hearted' this in school but it didn't quite touch your heart? Here's an example. Your grandmom told you that betel leaf is a great source of iron and you scoffed and figured that she comes up with excuses to validate her addiction to paan. Your child informs you that he will eat spinach today because Popeye says it's a rich source of iron. You weep and drown in tears of joy. You tweet that kids today are so smart, and so well-informed because of all the 'exposure' they receive, blah, blah.

The thing is, your grandmom is right and Popeye's spiel about iron is a myth. Betel leaf has five times more iron than spinach! Yeah, pick up your jaw. When you learnt all about digestion in your science class you also learnt that iron can't be absorbed without its co-factors, vitamin B and vitamin C. Betel leaf is an abundant source of these vitamins too, along with carotene, that's vitamin A, and has enzymes that aid digestion. Now you see why your grand old lady is chewing it post-lunch and has a memory of an elephant? She knows that chewing paan with lime, gulkand, clove, etc. (not tobacco) allows the secretion of enzymes required to absorb and assimilate the iron without loading her gastro-intestinal tract. Come on, go tweet about your grandmom's wisdom now!

Singhada

What is it?

The toast of winter, this aquatic vegetable is one of the many delicacies that i ate on my recent trip to Gadchiroli. It also grows naturally in ponds and lakes in many parts of central India. This nutrient-loaded food then is not just good for the people but also for the planet. The singhada is a winner and that could well be the reason for the seller's smile too.

Why to eat?

The water chestnut is a rich dose of antioxidants, minerals and vitamins. Traditionally, it is known to improve fertility levels (curtails growth of tumours and promotes hormonal balance), lower BP and offer relief from acidity.

It's one of the veggies that is recommended during fasts. And i am always touched by how all rituals of our culture, fasts included, promoted diversity in our diet.

How to eat?

You can eat it raw, just peel it open.

You could roast it, and then peel and eat.

You could dry it, make it into an atta and then make rotis out of it, which is popular during fasts.

It's a dessert, a mid-meal snack and a main meal. Every reason to eat it. Have you had one yet?

Tadgola

Just like the beauty of the rose, the juicy, madhur taste of the tadgola cannot be described in words. In Tamil culture, it's a tree of divine significance because it offers humanity everything we seek. Fruit to eat, neera to drink and even tadi to get high on. It's a fruit that can make you pregnant and can also be eaten during pregnancy. It can be eaten by your infant and your ninety-year-old grandmom. The fruit of the rich and of the poor.

In Maharashtra, the neera is a summer drink that delights and detoxes. Safe for all kinds of conditions—diabetes, liver, kidney or heart issues. Neera is the original virgin drink collected from the sap of the tree in the wee hours of the morning and drunk just around sunrise. If it will cleanse at sunrise, it will intoxicate at sundown.

The magical tree is even revered as a living goddess. It rises tall, demarcates one field from another and gives shade without overpowering the produce in the field.

Sadly, this tree is now facing neglect and the only ones left standing are the old trees. Young trees are not being planted and imported varieties of palm that bear no fruit, offer no shelter to bird, bees or butterflies are being used as decorative trees at airports and other landmarks across the country.

The pride in local starts with awareness. It also starts with what the young and educated put on their plates and plant in their gardens.

Metkut

Have you tried metkut yet? It's also known as buknu, menthittu or parupu poldi across India.

What is it?

A dry mixture of pulses and spices like haldi, soonth, etc.

How to eat it?

Sprinkle on hot rice, add ghee and enjoy. (Can also add it in curd and eat with bhakri/roti.)

Why?

When mixed with rice, it provides a complete amino acid profile in a no-fuss, easy preparation. Used as a substitute when you can't eat or don't feel like eating regular dal-rice.

Who can eat it?

1. Kids—especially in age group of two to five years. They naturally don't feel like eating dal-rice, and this is an age-old recipe to ensure they get all the nutrition they need. More details in my book, *Notes for Healthy Kids*.
2. Patients—for example, those suffering from chronic diseases or undergoing treatment for cancer. Their appetite goes for a toss but this is easy on the stomach and improves irritability and mood as well.
3. Everyone—after long travel or when suffering from constipation, or just for a change.

Let's bring the pulses back on our plate (at least twelve different pulses every year) and celebrate them in all their glory.

RECIPE FOR METKUT

Ingredients:

Rice, 1 katori
Urad dal, ½ katori
Chana dal, 2 katori
Coriander seeds, 2 teaspoons
Jeera, 1 teaspoon
Haldi powder, 1 teaspoon or halkund, 1 inch
Ajwain, ½ teaspoon
Soonth, ½ teaspoon
Red chillies, 2
Salt to taste

Steps:

- Dry roast the dals and rice.
- Grind the dal-rice mixture with all the other ingredients. Metkut is ready.
- Store in an airtight glass bottle.
- Sprinkle on hot mau bhat. Add ghee and enjoy.
- You can also add metkut to curd and eat with bhakri/roti.

Hyperlocal fruits

The 12 week fitness project 2020

Rujuta Diwekar

How are hyper-local fruits different from common local fruits

	Common local fruits	**Hyper local fruits**
What are they?	Commonly known and available seasonal fruits. Usually available across the country during season time.	Forgotten and not easily available fruits which are local to a particular region only. Also known as wild and uncultivated fruits or technically – NUS – neglected and underutilized species.
How to identify?	- Easily available in season with local vendors. - However, no advertisements or endorsements. - Usually misunderstood as not suitable for diabetes, weight loss, etc.	- No easy English name - Available for a very short time - Used to be sold outside schools and railway stations - Associated with folk tales, festivals, rituals, etc.
Examples	Banana, Mango, Chickoo, grapes, sitaphal, apple, guava, plum, peach, jackfruit, papaya, pomegranate, watermelon, muskmelon, pear, strawberry, lichi	Bora (ber), Maran (coconut flower), Phalsa (local berry), Shehtooth (mulberry), Karvanda , Ranjana, Jamun, Bel, Cashew fruit, Dhurchuk (Seabuckthorn), Tadgola, Fresh dates, Nimboli (neem fruit), Kamrakh (star fruit), Ramphal
Why to eat?	- Full of nutrients and a good prebiotic - Keeps the local economy chugging - Often also turned into pickles, jams, candies, etc.	- Supports tribal and marginalized communities - Help with the micro-nutrient deficiencies - Supports gut function
When to eat?	- As a mid-meal - When main meals are delayed - Sometimes with main meal also	- As mid-meals while the 2-3-week window lasts

Section Three

FOOD IS MEDICINE

“

RUJUTA SAYS...

Low-fat and low-calorie will invariably lead to low vitamin D, the deficiency of which is a known risk for cancer. Get fit, not thin.

Rice, ghee, kaju to calm the nerves and the heart. Along with strength training to strengthen the heart muscle. Strong and happy heart = fearless, joyful life. :-)

Spend more time in farms to spend less money on pharms.

Before taking those vitamin D ‘shots’, give ghee a chance. One teaspoon at breakfast, lunch and dinner and say tata to weak bones and pigmented skin.

Immunity is not a genie that comes out of a bottle, it’s a natural response of the human body.

Wine is very good for the heart of the person who doesn’t drink it. #worldheartday

”

3A. FOODS FOR COMMON HEALTH CONDITIONS

PCOD/Thyroid issues

Top three guidelines for PCOD

1. The real indicators of health: Use your natural intelligence and not AI or scales to gauge your health. The three most important indicators are:
i) Energy levels through the day.
ii) Quality of sleep during the night.
iii) Compliance to exercise plan.

2. Super foods for PCOD: A diverse diet is key to maintaining diverse gut bacteria, which in turn helps with insulin sensitivity and regulates periods.
i) Coconut, ghee, jaggery and aliv seeds help with enlarged pores on the skin.
ii) Raw banana, suran, sprouted legumes prevent PMS and migraine, also prevent spotting that goes on for days together.
iii) Nachni, either as dosa, porridge or bhakri, prevents cramps and acne that comes around the chin.

3. For a pain-free period:
i) Weight train once a week to improve bone mineral density and muscle tone.
ii) Practice yoga asanas, especially the restorative poses like supta baddha konasana to ease pain during heavy flow.
iii) Take a calcium and B12 supplement during the entire week of the period to keep cramps and head/back aches at bay.

RECIPE FOR SPROUTED MOONG

Ingredients:

Mung, ½ katori

Ghee, 1 teaspoon

Curd, 1 katori

Saindha namak

Green chillies, chopped fine

Dhania

Steps:

- Sprout mung.
- Place in a steel pot, add some water and the ghee.
- Cook in a pressure cooker.
- Because of the ghee, the mung will not get overcooked. (In fact, you can cook other sprouts in ghee also without it getting overcooked).
- Once cooked, add the curd, namak, green chilli.
- Mix and add fresh dhania

Q & A on PCOD and thyroid issues

Q. Has the conversation around PCOD changed in the last decade?

Yes! Since 2005, we've started seeing more and more people get diagnosed with PCOD and thyroid issues. Earlier, people would approach me with problems regarding weight loss. Those were the initial conversations. Now, since 2011, people have been coming up to me with problems like 'i don't think i can get pregnant'—and this came from a girl in the 9th grade. So, the conversation around PCOD has changed. It has become about fear;

it has become another way of making women feel really inadequate in their body and about what they would be capable of doing later on.

So the diagnosis is also getting very aggressive. But there are a whole lot of things that one can do to deal with it. Starting from what you eat, what time you sleep, and committing to regular exercise. So many of these things are in our hands. It's a matter of a few months or a year, a year and a half in extreme cases, before you can lead a completely hormonally happy life.

Q. What are the warning signs that we need to watch out for?

The warning sign that we really need to watch out for is basically how much we're sitting. If we're sitting for hours and hours together, then that's the first warning sign. Because a sedentary lifestyle is the first step towards what is known as 'insulin resistance', where our insulin doesn't function as optimally as it is supposed to function. And that is the root cause for PCOD, thyroid issues and diabetes too. Instead of looking for symptoms on the outside like 'Am i getting fat?', 'Am i not fitting into my jeans?', all you really need to do is pay attention to signs of a lifestyle that exposes you to these lifestyle diseases.

Q. Is there a particular age group that is more prone to these ailments?

i think typically, in India, it's when girls are studying for 12th grade exams, or when they start living in a hostel where there aren't any home-cooked meals or for that matter when they take up a job that changes their lifestyle, where all of a sudden they have accessible income and they start eating things that are more expensive but not necessarily rich in terms of nutrients. So, at any point when you experience an erratic lifestyle, women tend to become susceptible to things like PCOD and thyroid issues. And basic things like eating outside food, sitting for too long and being exposed to stress are all major factors.

Q. Monitoring your weight is extremely important when you're dealing with PCOD. What is the best form of exercise that women should be getting?

First things first, it's not body weight that is important. What is very, very important is body composition. And the reason is that the more muscle tissue you lose, the more insulin resistant you get. And when the body gets insulin-resistant, you will start putting on weight, develop pigmentation, break-out, etc. In this whole journey of losing weight, what we tend to do is adopt methods that compromise our muscle tissue. That's what most crash diets and fads do. So the best form of exercise that one can do is strength training in the gym regularly, because it can rebuild lost muscle tissue.

Q. Five lifestyle changes one should make to keep PCOS and thyroid issues in control?

If you've been sitting for thirty minutes, stand for at least three minutes.

Eat homemade food. Bring back ghee, curd, rice. Basically everything your grandmother endorses.

Always fix what you're going to eat between 4 and 6 p.m. a week before. Because that's the time that we tend to mess up the most, and we land up eating everything that we never wanted to eat.

Adopt 150 minutes of weekly exercises as a way of life.

Get rid of your gadgets at least an hour before you hit the bed.

Q. The biggest health myth out there?
That you must lose weight to get healthy. And that soups and salads are healthier than dal and rice.
Q. The one food that you should be eating that no one is talking about?
Kokum. It's a coastal food. You can make a sherbet out of it and it works really well to keep acidity at bay and tackles all the other extra problems that come with PCOD and thyroid issues, like bloating, headaches, etc. So it's a great food to add to your diet.

Top three foods—thyroid problems

- Fresh fruit of the season daily.
- Dry coconut as a snack.
- A millet for dinner.

Will help with:

- Hypothyroidism
- Blood sugar regulation
- Joint issues
- Infertility

PMS/ Period pain

Five foods for PMS/Period pain

Include these five foods to reduce the aches, pain, cramps, migraine, nausea, mood-swings, etc., during PMS or period pain.

1. Soaked raisins and kesar first thing in morning, at least a week before periods.
2. Ghee with all meals.
3. Dahi-rice with legumes for lunch with fried papad.
4. Handful of peanuts or cashews as mid-meal.
5. Khichdi or rajgeera or kuttu for dinner.

A full-day meal plan for periods

Follow this for a week before periods and till the last day of periods. If you're not sure about your period date, start following when you experience PMS symptoms. These suggestions are for everyone with reproductive health issues and cover most symptoms before or after periods.

Use this as a reference and adapt it to your region and availability. Eat as per appetite.

Rujuta Diwekar

The Period Plan

- Follow it for a week before periods and till the last day of periods
- If not sure about your period date, start following when you experience PMS symptoms
- These suggestions are for everyone with reproductive health issues and cover most symptoms before or after periods
- Use this as a reference and adapt it to your region and availability. Eat as per appetite.

Meal Timings	**Meal options**	**Comments**
Within 15 mins of waking up	Overnight soaked raisins (6-7) + soaked strands of kesar (1-2)	-Have banana also in case of migraines and constipation
Breakfast (within 60-90 mins of M1)	Any homemade breakfast- Sabudana khichdi/ Any stuffed paratha with white butter/ Rajgeera sheera/ Sama ke chawal kheer	- Can have your tea/coffee with breakfast
Mid-meal (within 2-3 hours of breakfast)	Coconut + jaggery/ Jaggery + whole 2-3 dhaniya seeds/ Any fresh seasonal sherbet/ Coconut water	- Follow the Iyengar yoga restorative asanas at least 3 days a week
Lunch (latest by 1.30pm)	Rice or roti + sabzi + dal + ghee + dahi or pickle or papad or chutney OR Dahi rice with achaar or papad or steamed sprouts	-Sabzi- yam/ arbi/ any gourd/ pumpkin/ raw banana, etc., 4 days/ week -Pulses (sprouted & cooked)- lobia, moong, masur, kulith, chana, rajma, etc., 4 days/week
Evening snack (between 4-6pm)	Aliv ladoo or aliv kheer/Boiled sweet potato with rock salt or kees/ Arbi or suran kaap/ seasonal fruit/ handful of cashews & jaggery	-Make your traditional snack of arbi or sweet potato - Don't have tea/coffee post 5 pm - Suptabadhakonasana for 10-15 mins
Dinner (2-3 hours before bedtime)	Any rice preparation with paneer/ Rice pej with deep fried papad/ Curd rice with tadka/ Khichdi + ghee + achaar or papad or raita or kadhi	
At bedtime (if hungry, before sleeping)	1 tsp of gulkand/ banana	-Vipareet karni inversion before periods (stop when periods begin)

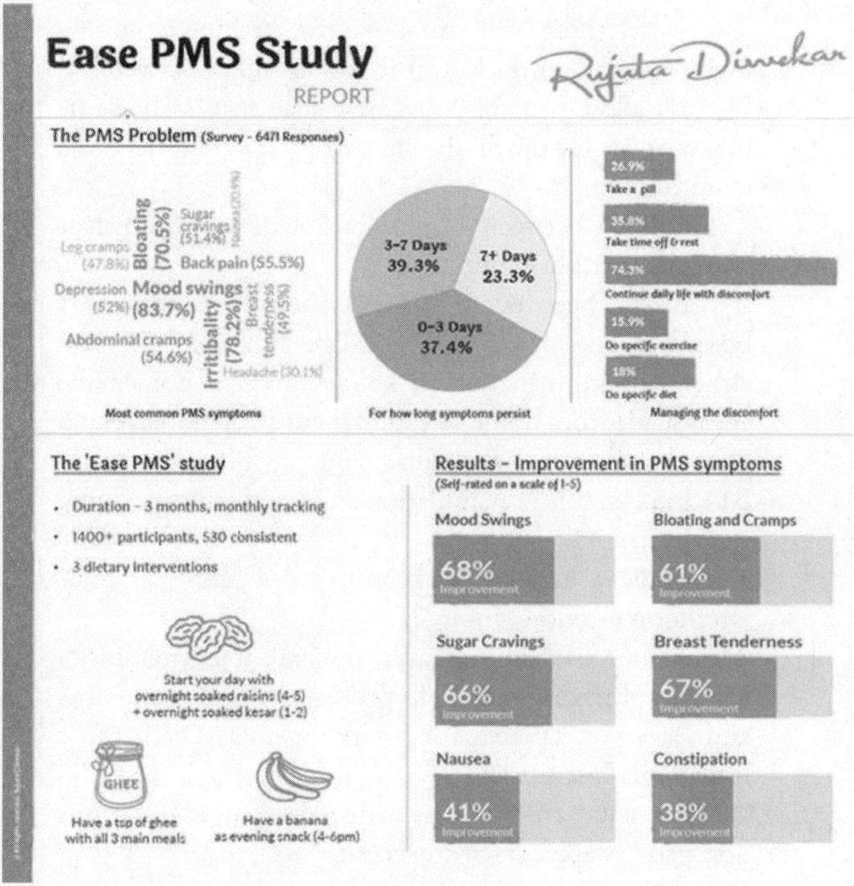

Diabetes

Five easy tips for diabetics to regulate your blood sugars better

1. Start your day with a fresh, seasonal fruit or banana or soaked and peeled badam.

The worst thing you can do is to go hungry post a night of fasting or kick-start it with a cup of chai/coffee. Instead, allow your body its best chance to stabilise its blood sugars for the day by starting with a fresh fruit or a handful of nuts.

2. Eat lunch between 11 a.m. and 1 p.m. and finish it with chaas or buttermilk.

If you have been taking diabetic meds for a while, it's bound to take a toll on your digestion and leave you either with constipation or IBS. A glass of homemade chaas made from home-set, full-fat curd will not just help your digestion but also allow you to optimise vitamin B12 and vitamin D assimilation and kill the sugar craving post lunch.

3. Include a handful of peanuts as a snack for mid-afternoon or mid-evening.

A rich source of amino acids, minerals and vitamins, a handful of peanuts can help protect the heart and joints and leave you satiated for hours together. Ditch those fibre-waala biscuits.

4. When you have chai, one teaspoon of sugar is fine but don't add sweeteners or stevia.

Diabetes is often reduced to a high blood sugar problem but the real danger is that of the cells starving and the complications of heart, kidney, neuromuscular issues that may arise out of that. A teaspoon of sugar is a safer bet than artificial sweeteners or even stevia, as these often lead to higher circulating levels of insulin, which further increases your insulin resistance. So, max two–three cups of chai or coffee in a day, and use cane sugar and full fat milk.

5. Weight train at least twice a week.
Cannot emphasise this enough (and will probably make a video on this soon), but loss of muscular strength is one of the drivers of insulin resistance. Strength training done in the gym with weights or even at home with resistance bands can help reverse insulin resistance. So get your dose of exercise; it will help you cut back on the drug dosages dramatically. Medical advice is notoriously slow to catch up with the latest in exercise science, but know that if your doctor is allowing you to walk, you are good to gym too. Use the beginner's plan from *Don't Lose Out Work Out!*

Top five myths about diabetes

1. Avoid banana but apple is okay.
All fruits contain natural sugars, mostly fructose, which has a low glycaemic index. Banana is even approved by the American Diabetes Association, but shunned by doctors and dietitians in the country of its origin. Banana is not just safe but recommended for people with diabetes as it is mineral-rich and helps prevent high BP too.
2. Avoid sugar in chai/coffee but biscuits like Marie and digestive are okay.
That teaspoon or even two of sugar in your chai is much better than the low-grade sugar, trans-fat and emulsifier-rich biscuit/cracker. The thing is, if you see sugar as a problem, you may continue having your chai/coffee/cola without sugar. If you must beat diabetes, then you must see that the real risk comes from unregulated intake of food and misinformation about what is good or bad for

you. So have the chai with sugar but limit it to max two to three cups a day, and don't touch biscuits and the likes.

3. Ghee specifically and fat in general must be avoided.

Nothing could be further away from the truth. Addition of fat lowers the rate at which blood sugars climb and don't overburden insulin (the hormone responsible for blood sugar regulation). Ghee and coconut both have the essential fatty acids that further support insulin, protect the heart and help maintain the intestinal mucosa. So if you are diabetic, the one thing that you can't afford to miss out on is fat, and more specifically, ghee. Eat loads of it.

4. Walking is the best exercise, cardio is good.

Lift weights and join a gym. Train your big muscles and develop strength in them as loss of strength from the body is directly linked to insulin resistance and incidence of diabetes. If you are diabetic, gymming is the best exercise for you.

5. Once you are diabetic, you stay diabetic.

Not true. It's easy to regulate blood sugars and support insulin function through the right approach to diet, exercise and lifestyle. It's important though to take it a step at a time. Medical journals are slowly but steadily waking up to the fact that their diet guidelines have been way off the mark and that eating traditional, local and seasonal is one of the easiest and most inexpensive ways to stay healthy.

We have been systematically taken away from our native eating habits and introduced to new ones to live healthier lives. But in the bargain we have gotten fatter, sicker and diabetic. It's never too late to change though. Start small, start with the basics: work out, eat the way your grandmom taught you to and regulate your bedtime. Your stress and sugars both will climb down and your confidence will climb up.

World Diabetes Day from the chirota's point of view

Hello friends. Not a very happy Diwali for me, if you are asking who's chirota. Don't look up Google, there's no English name for me, i am a native just like you. The reason why i am writing is that, just like native plants and fruits, no one seems to care that i am about to go extinct. If i were an animal, the WWF would put me on that critically endangered list. i am grateful for the long life i have had; i have seen the world go by and maybe it's just age (though my creator promised me that i was ageless like Bheeshma), but i am beginning to understand that no one quite cares about us native, traditional sweets. Not the governments, no right-wing group, no leftist, no atheist, and of course no chef, dietitian or doctor.

The reason for my critically endangered status is the exact same thing that makes us a diabetic nation—misinformation. And misinformation repeated multiple times by doctors, dietitians, etc., till it becomes the truth. And it's not just me, i am just one sweet from Maharashtra, but there are many like me across every region in India and i am not even counting the ones across the rest of the developing world who join me in this plight. But then every truth must be questioned before being accepted.

So i am my own voice and i want you to hear the truth. If you are reading this on a laptop, phone, computer, you didn't need me, free internet should have allowed you to have all this information, but here goes:

1. Food is not the sum total of carbs, protein and fat, there's much more there than meets the eye. And nutrition science is taking its own sweet time to get there.
2. Sugar is not the problem, nor is it the solution—you are. If you drink sugarless tea with a biscuit in your hand (however tasteless the biscuit) you are just clueless. The American Diabetes Association says that roughly about six to nine teaspoons of sugar a day is healthy. Now trust me, even by chirota standards that's too much. With that much sugar, i can feed six of you a super-size me each.
3. Addition of fat, especially the good old ghee, delays gastric emptying by up-regulating the response of a gut hormone called GLP-1. Adding ghee to food, in this case adding it to maida, lowers the glycaemic index of maida, which on its own has a pretty high GI. Whether its hormonal imbalance, obesity or diabetes that you are fighting, adding ghee to your diet is a great idea.

So really, Diwali deserves to be celebrated with us native sweets that bring families and societies together, and that's not something that chocolates, cupcakes and mindlessly re-cycled gifts can ever do.

Where will you find a chirota?

Not at any fancy store, not when you unwrap fancy packing, it's now made by small women's groups or cooperatives. So until you learn to make a chirota at home, know that every time you buy a chirota, you keep a woman in business, a child in school and a family financially able to celebrate Diwali!

Heart health/Cholesterol

Easy tips for a healthy heart

1. Switch back to kacche ghani ka groundnut, mustard, til, coconut oil—retains micronutrients and delicate carbon bonds in fatty acids, helps fight free radicals that damage the heart.
2. Eat ghee in every meal—regulates postprandial blood sugar response.
3. Have homemade pickle or moramba (especially of amla and other forgotten berries) or chutneys (of til/curry patta/flaxseed/peanut/garlic)—adds value to the meal and cuts down on sugar cravings and bloating.
4. Exercise 150 minutes every week + at least one day of strength training in the gym. Lowers resting heartrate, improves quality of life.
5. Sleep and wake up at a fixed time every day and make time for a twenty-minute nap post lunch. Improves recovery and digestion. An undervalued aspect of heart health.
6. Lastly, dil pe mat lo. Forget, forgive, forward.

Top four points jo dil dhadkaenge at right time for right reasons and not coz of anger and stress

1. Eat food based on what's grown locally and not based on calories. E.g., local fruits have the same fructose as the exotic ones, and in addition have nutrients we need. So

have banana, chickoo, mango, grapes. The demand for these fruits will also lead to farmers' wellbeing.

2. Eat ghee, kaju, coconut and kacha ghani seed oils. The addition of fat decreases the glycaemic index of food and they don't have any adverse effect on cholesterol production. Refined vegetable oils are now linked to increased incidences of heart disease.

3. Take the effort to find hand-pounded rice rather than wasting time trying to cook brown rice. Rice-pounding is the extra effort taken to remove the husk so that optimum fibre, vitamin B and zinc—which improve insulin sensitivity—are accessible. If not hand-pounded, get single-polished rice.

4. Listen to your stomach to know how much to eat and when to stop—keep phones, TV, newspaper away while eating.

Apne pet ki awaz apne dil aur dimag mai utaro.

Truth about cholesterol

- Avoiding 'cholesterol' by choosing 'low fat' options only leads to lower levels of vitamin D and sex hormones.
- Egg yolk is a good source of essential fatty acid DHA (omega 3). Still wanna avoid yolk and pop an omega 3 pill?
- The misunderstood cholesterol is a critical nutrient without which your liver cannot produce bile, the substance which allows our body to digest and process fat.
- Rich in medium chain triglycerides, coconut reduces bloating, overeating and risk to cholesterol and heart diseases.

• Cashews have copper that keeps blood vessels flexible, which improves lipid profile and reduces hypercholesterolemia.

• High levels of cholesterol and low vitamin D go together. Ghee in your meals will help you lower LDL and improve vitamin D assimilation.

Cancer

Nutrition during and after cancer treatment

(Summary of my talk at Tata Memorial Hospital, Mumbai on 5 February 2020)

Part 1: Foods to have during and after cancer treatment (chemo, radiation, etc.) to counter acidity, low energy, irritability, weakness, indigestion, lack of sleep, loss of appetite, hair loss, etc.

• Gulkand—mix a teaspoon in water and sip it during the day. Effective for acidity and burning sensation during the treatment. Have it with milk in the night when you are having sleeplessness. Good for constipation also.

• Rice—effective when you don't feel like eating anything. Also helps with irritability.

a) Kanji or pej: liquid form of rice; retains more nutrients than vegetable soups. You can add ghee to it.

b) Metkut rice: add metkut mixture (dry dal and herbs) to rice to get a complete protein profile. (Instead of having rice with dal, as sometimes patients don't feel like having dal.) Add ghee. Especially good for small kids.

• Home-set curd: good source of B12 and helps with Hb production. For kids, when setting dahi, add four to five black raisins. This way you can eat it as a mid-meal snack also. Also effective for old people and for women with low Hb.

• Chaas: hand-churned chaas (back and forth action) and not in a mixer or with spoon. This way it retains all nutrients. Good for the intestinal mucosa and lining of the stomach which often gets compromised during treatment. With chaas, add three things—kala namak + jeera + hing. Good for acidity/burning sensation. Also nourishes the taste buds and will bring back the appetite.

• Amla: as muramba, sherbet or pickle. Good source of vitamin C and B12 and helps in Hb production. Also works as an antacid. Make it now and use it through the year.

• Aliv: as aliv laddoo for strength in the body. Good source of iron and folic acid. Eat it three to four days post chemo. It's also effective for removing skin dullness and darkening and aids hair growth.

• Nachni/ragi: for headache, mental fog, weak bones, etc. It's a good source of calcium and micro minerals. Have as nachni pej or kheer during treatment (when acidity is high) and later as bhakri, etc.

Part 2: What not to do during treatment

Don't follow WhatsApp diets. For example:

• Green juices (raw vegetable juices) like wheatgrass, palak, methi, etc. Green vegetables are healthy but only when eaten after cooking with tadka, etc.

• Heating coconut water before drinking. Have it as we normally do and in small quantities. Have tadgola also.

• Haldi, jeera or ajwain shots. These spices are effective in small quantities when used as part of cooking. If we have them in water, it will interfere with nutrient assimilation. Too much haldi will reduce levels of iron also.

• Fasting. Eating on time will make the treatment effective and also prevent headaches, irritability and weakness.

Part 3: For caregivers

First acknowledge that you are doing a very difficult job and don't put too much pressure on yourself. Pay attention to your health as it effects the health of the patient too.

• Three meals you must have: a) don't go to the hospital on an empty stomach, have a fresh fruit or a simple homemade nashta b) have lunch between 12 and 1 p.m. Don't delay it to 3–4 p.m. c) between 4–6 p.m., eat a wholesome meal. Helps with regulating cortisol.

• Good option to bring with you when you accompany the patient for treatment is roti with ghee and jaggery. Other options—phodni cha bhaat (rice with tadka). Even phodni chi roti or chura.

• Exercise/activity is important. For both patients and caregivers. Even a small amount of time spent in being active helps. For caregivers, try and do two to three surynamaskars every day.

To summarise: It's important to eat well to recover, to make the treatment effective and keep the side-effects in check.

RUJUTA SAYS...

Secret to a flat stomach—hop, skip, jump and not just crunch.

The only way to develop a flat stomach is through strength, more specifically strength in your legs, and not reduction in your calories.

Kokum over quinoa, kela over kiwi and local over low-cal to reduce waste (ecological) and waist. Also to broaden your smile and mind.

Dear instant noodles, health cannot be built in two minutes even if you add vegetables to it. ;-)

Fruit crisps instead of real chips, baked over fried, yucky over yummy, is not healthy just silly.

Hunger is a sign of youth, don't suppress it.

3B. QUICK TIPS FOR GOOD HEALTH

Home exercise and diet—HEAD project

The HEAD start project

Home exercise and diet

Rujuta Diwekar

Diet Rules	Details
1. Don't start your day with tea/coffee	- Have something to eat, like dry fruits or a fresh fruit after waking up and then have tea/coffee. - Limit tea/ coffee to 3 cups a day. Have them the way you like it, with sugar, milk, masala, etc. - Don't have tea/coffee as a replacement to a meal or post evening (4-5pm)
2. Finish your dinner 3 hours before bedtime	- Don't push bedtime late, bring dinner early - If you are hungry at bedtime, have haldi-milk or gulkand with milk
3. Avoid long gaps between meals	- Homemade sherbet like Bel, Nimbu, Kokum, etc., between breakfast and lunch - Have something wholesome like a fresh fruit, handful of nuts or homemade nashta between lunch and dinner.
4. Finish eating your meals just before you are full	- Follow the 3 S of eating right to help you finish your meals at the right time – **Sit** – sit down at one fixed place to eat your meals. **Senses** – use your hands, chew well, and don't get distracted with gadgets/ TV. **Slow** – take your time to eat your meals so that you can listen to the signals from your stomach
5. Have ghee, fresh fruit and homemade chutney/pickle daily	- Ghee adds satiety and aids digestion. - Fresh, local, seasonal fruits provide all the nutrients needed by the body - Chutney/ pickle add all the micro-nutrients that body needs e.g. Vit b12, Vit K.
Exercise Rules	**Details**
1. Follow a well-rounded fitness regime	The 4S of Fitness – Strength, Stability, Stretching, Stamina Pay special attention to strength, stability and stretching as these are usually overlooked and only stamina is worked on.
2. Progressive overload principle	- Make gradual increase in the challenge level of the exercise - Continuity of practice is critical for staying fit

Gharelu nuskhe for cough, cold and flu

Here is a quick list:

1. Ghee, dry ginger powder (soonth), haldi, jaggery—mix in equal amounts, roll into nail-size balls, and eat first thing in the morning and last thing in the night.
2. Breakfast—ragi porridge or dosa.
3. Mid-morning—cashews + jaggery.
3. Lunch—moong dal with rice and ghee, every day.
4. Evening snack—jaggery, poha and milk or egg with toast or home-set curd and poha.
5. Dinner—dal khichdi or fish and rice or kulith (horse gram) pithla with rice and ghee.
6. Special drink—ginger, lemon, lemon grass and honey chai or like a Kashmiri kawah with kesar, ginger and almonds. Anytime during the day.

The time-tested wisdom from our kitchens and grandmoms shouldn't need a pandemic to come back into the limelight. Local ingredients, seasonal produce, spices and ghee have been the backbone of our food traditions, especially when one is under the weather or recovering from a flu. So dig in, chew it slowly and pass it on to the next generation. And do it exactly like your grandma did—with love.

How to fight cough, cold and chest congestion this winter

Before you pop an antibiotic, give time-tested, home-grown wisdom a chance. Do the following:

1. Mix methi dana (fenugreek) + jaggery + soonth (dry ginger powder), add it to milk and drink it.
2. If you also have the flu, add haldi + kesar to the above mixture.

3. Do the following sequence of asanas (only if you regularly practice yoga asanas):

- Sarvangasana
- Halasana
- Paschimottanasana

Alternative to having milk: soonth, gul and ghee ke small laddoo. Take equal amounts of dry ginger, jaggery and ghee, mix it well and roll it into small balls. Start and end your day with one. Also helpful to have one after you have returned home after spending a long time outdoors.

Top three foods that keep the digestion healthy during the shaadi season

1. Glass of chaas with hing and kala namak right after lunch. While the chaas or buttermilk is both a good source of probiotics and vitamin B12, the hing and kala namak combo will help cut down bloating, gas and even prevent IBS. Have it especially if you are attending evening functions and want to sport a flat stomach.
2. One teaspoon of chyawanprash at bedtime. Keeps the immune system strong and is a solid source of flavonoids and antioxidants, which will ensure that the skin stays supple and soft even through the torture of the wedding festivities. Have it if late-night shaadis are a routine and especially if you are at a destination wedding.
3. Methi laddoo made with jaggery, ghee and dry ginger. Prevents stomach cramps and constipation, promotes intestinal mucosa and even helps keep the hair lustrous, which can otherwise look frizzy due to a poorly

functioning stomach. Have it either at breakfast or as a 4–6 p.m. meal if your sleep routine has been disrupted and you are even missing workouts. Helps with blood sugar regulation too.

Top three tips for the alluring shaadi glow

Losing weight is something we would like because we want to look our best, and by that we mean at our thinnest. But have we really thought this through? At what cost do we really want to lose weight? Is thinner necessarily prettier? Does it really empower you to wear 'whatever you want'?

If we do use our brain then we realise that what really looks good on us is confidence and good health. That's all that we need to look our best, not just on D-day but day after day.

Here are the top three foods that you must have all the time, especially for three months before your D-day, to reap their full benefits.

1. Shudh desi ghee: The same one that your grandmom irritates you about. She's told you all the benefits, all i can say is that the grand old lady who defies her age has a point and you ought to be listening. You should have it because:

• It helps the mucus lining of the intestines, thereby reducing the chances of bloating. Especially the one that comes with late-night eating and sleepless nights. Now i would expect that thanks to all the late-night romantic calls.

• The essential fatty acids in ghee lead to good assimilation of fat-soluble vitamins, more specifically vitamin E, and add that touch of glow to your face.
• Increases the flavour of food and therefore satiety—helps auto-reduce the portion size of every meal and the calories consumed.

Tip: Have three to five teaspoons of ghee every day, preferably with meals.

2. Good old haldi: You don't need me to sell you this idea, in all probability you are also going to have a haldi function. There are reasons why haldi is so celebrated—it helps you get off that soup-salad regime and have regular dal-chawal-sabzi for dinner. And you do want to eat that haldi because:
• It is known for its ability to bust both physical and mental stress, and trust me you are going to need it.
• Prevents infections, and no one wants to land up with a urinary tract or vaginal infection ever, but surely not close to the wedding day.
• Here's an aesthetic reason—it helps the skin beat the effects of tannin and pigmentation and allows you to put your best face forward.

Tip: Use turmeric in daily cooking, and preferably buy it from a small women's organisation to reap its full benefits.

3. Home-set, full-fat dahi and chaas: i said home-set and full fat because i don't want you buying packaged yoghurt or a fat-free version. The beauty lies in the fat, and without it, the curd is not of much use.
• It's the tastiest and easiest way to provide your body

with gut-friendly bacteria. It not only reduces bloating but actually gives the stomach a flat look.

• A good source of minerals like calcium, it helps strengthen bone density and gives you a good toned versus flabby look.

• India's favourite digestive aid, it will actually allow you to metabolise the food that you are eating. Oral wisdom also says that it lets you metabolise or digest tough situations, and wedding season offers you more than one tough situation. So bring on the lassi.

Tip: Have at least a few teaspoons of dahi before stepping out for long shopping hours and parties. It will reduce the acidity that follows. Better still, carry chaas with you in a flask.

i wish you a long and healthy life and partnership with Mr Right.

The top five Indian food secrets that will help you kill cellulite

Almost everyone is worried about stretch marks/cellulite. Almost everyone thinks that there is no cure. Almost everyone has spent money on creams/oils/gels that don't really help. And almost everyone has ignored the open secrets from the Indian kitchen that actually help prevent cellulite and even get rid of existing ones.

So here are the top five Indian foods to get rid of cellulite:

1. Kharvas/cheekh/bari or colostrum: Rich in antibodies and growth factors like IGF-1, it not only helps burn fat

but also works at visibly reducing stretch marks from the skin.

2. Kokum: Has made it to UN's list of NUS (Neglected and Underutilised Species) for its multiple nutritional benefits, but more relevant for us here is the HCA, hydroxy citric acid, that prevents lipogenesis, i.e. build-up of fat stores.

3. Ghee: No list of Indian foods can be complete without it. Rich in SCFA (short chain fatty acid) and butyric acid, it prevents inflammation of not just the intestines but all the tissues of the body, and ensures that nothing pops out of that smooth skin of yours.

4. Banana flower: Rich in enzymes and its ability to strike the right hormonal balance (especially in women), it ensures that stretch marks don't even begin to appear on your body. No wonder it enjoys the reputation of preventing menstrual pain and excess bleeding (hormonal balance).

5. Kesar: Celebrated the world over for its ability to give you a smooth skin and glowing complexion, kesar is rich in aromatic volatile compounds that help keep the free radicals (metabolites that can cause skin damage or ageing) under check. P.S.: it's also the secret therapy for premature ejaculation.

Khaddi shakkar

Ayurveda has celebrated the khaddi shakkar, or misri as it is called, for centuries and celebrated its therapeutic value for easing a cough, preventing a cold and strengthening a weak immune system.

It is also popular with Indian classical singers to keep their vocal chords lucid, fluid and sweet.

It's also known to keep acidity, nausea and gas down.

As for all those of you who worry about 'sugar', know that what you need to avoid are the ultra-processed, packaged foods like biscuits, colas and chocolates. The misri is medicinal, and when taken as a part of a healthy, wholesome diet and a disciplined lifestyle, works wonders. Bite into it yet?

Immunity-boosting is the new weight loss

There's an industry waiting to launch products, pills and potions to monetise on your fears and insecurities. If it was weight loss yesterday, it's going to be immunity tomorrow. But don't forget that good health begins at home. So:

- cook often
- care for your family
- common sense will always see you through

Dengue—prevention and recovery

One of the main reasons for the increased incidences of dengue (i am told it's pronounced as dengee) in our lives today is, of course, more mosquitoes, but also the fact that people have weaker immune systems.

Constant dieting and over-exercising often puts people at risk, so does having unregulated blood sugars and hormonal imbalances (read PCOD, diabetes and thyroid issues).

Here's a list of things that are both tasty and therapeutic—they go a long way in preventing the risk of infection and accelerate recovery:

1. One teaspoon of gulkand either first thing in the morning or between meals. Prevents acidity, nausea and weakness.
2. One glass of milk + one glass of water, add a pinch of haldi, two–three strands of kesar, a tiny bit of jaiphal (nutmeg)—boil this till it's half the quantity. Add jaggery to taste and have it cold or hot. Boosts immunity, reduces inflammation and prevents protein loss.
3. Rice kanji or pej—essentially a soup made of rice. Add kala namak or sendha namak, a pinch of hing (try and get the good one from Kochi) and ghee. Prevents dehydration, loss of electrolytes and works on improving appetite.
4. Water—sip on it through the day to restore urine volume and check that the colour is clear.
5. Practice supta badha konasana, the Iyengar style, with a bolster to support the back and a blanket under your head if needed to support the neck. Helps relieve backache and body pains, allows the trunk to relax.

Foods for NRIs

NRIs Health Series Rujuta Diwekar

Most common problems	What to eat	Habits to follow
- Acidity/ bloating - Indigestion - Weight gain - Acne and patchy skin - Hair fall and dry scalp Why? - Change in diet, climate, timings, schedule, etc. - Gut bacteria diversity goes for a toss.	- Non-perishables from your heritage/ culture - Perishables from local Non-perishables – Grains, pulses, millets, spices, oils. Use traditional cooking methods. Perishables – Fruits, vegetables, dairy, meat. Support farmers market.	- Avoid long gaps between meals. - Replace one of the tea/coffee with nimbu sherbet/ buttermilk/ laban. - Talk about food in your mother tongue. - Include atleast one day of strength training every week and daily yoga asana - Fix your bedtime. Don't stay up late as it effects hormonal balance.
Foods for good digestion	**Foods for skin and hair**	**Foods that last long**
1. Banana 2. Curd rice 3. Ghee 4. Pickle 5. Local vegetables	1. Dry coconut 2. Til/ sesame 3. Aliv seeds 4. Rajgeera 5. Sprouted pulses	1. Chiwda 2. Ragi laddoos 3. Red pumpkin puri 4. Curry leaves chutney 5. Metkut (mix of dals, spices)

Simple home tips to beat the smog

1. Soonth, gul and ghee ke bite-size laddoo. Take equal amounts of dry ginger, jaggery and ghee, mix it well, and roll it into small balls. Start and end your day with one. Also helpful to have one after spending a long time outdoors.

- Prevents inflammation and flu.
- Keeps sinuses clear.
- Helps digestion.

2. Sugarcane—either chew on it and spit the fibre out (in the correct places, of course) or drink it like a fresh juice. Preferably mid-meal, eaten before noon.

- Cleanses and helps detoxify the liver.
- Micronutrient-dense, so boosts the immune system.
- Helps beat lethargy and low moods due to smog.

3. Milk, kesar, haldi and soaked sabja as a nightcap. Heat milk, and add kesar and haldi while it's still on the boil. Add one teaspoon of soaked sabja or tulsi seeds after you pour it in a cup; you can also add powdered jaggery to taste.

- Volatile oils from kesar prevent skin and hair damage.
- Sabja or tulsi seeds beat infections, allergies and bloating.
- Haldi + milk is a potent and well-known recovery and anti-inflammatory combo.

Other tips:

- Don't give up on exercise, just shift it indoors.
- Stay well hydrated.
- Vitamin D, vitamin B12 and carotene supplements are helpful in these situations.

Home remedies for dark circles

1. Stay away from toxic people both online and offline.
2. Make a chai of ginger, tulsi, kesar, add honey and drink once a day.
3. Mix a little bit of peanuts, jaggery and coconut in a bowl and enjoy it as a 4 p.m. snack.

4. Learn to do the halasana with the spine aligned.
5. Mix besan and fresh milk to make a paste and use it as a cleanser for the face. Avoid soaps/face wash.

Top five foods to keep the acne away

1. Cashew fruit: Five times the vitamin C than an orange, this one is filled with minerals that kill pimples even before they arrive.
Eat—mid-afternoon snack.
2. Jackfruit: The immunity booster that regulates hormones and ensures that testosterone is kept under check, it leaves the skin looking flawless.
Eat—anytime in the day.
3. Nariyal pani: Hydrates and has the electrolyte balance to help the body flush out all that is causing toxicity.
Eat—anytime before noon.
4. Gulkand: Antibacterial and antiviral, it boosts the gut bacteria and helps get rid of marks that acne leaves behind.
Eat—half a teaspoon post lunch and dinner.
5. Aliv (garden cress): Iron- and mineral-rich source, which when mixed with jaggery and coconut will not just give you a glowing complexion but boost energy levels too.
Eat—mid-meal anytime of the day.

Top 3 foods for common health problems

Rujuta Diwekar

(bit.ly/top3foodsrujuta)

Health issue	**Common in**	**Top 3 foods**			**Special tip**
Constipation	Diabetes BP PCOD Insomnia PMS	**Jaggery + ghee** - Have it post lunch	Any local **melon** – 3-4 pm meal in summers	Add **Til** to roti/ bhakri at dinner	Stay well hydrated.
Thyroid issues	Hypothyroid Joint-problems Blood sugar Infertility	**Mango or banana** – Anytime but esp. with lunch	**Dry coconut** – by itself or as chutney or with snack – Pre-workout	**Kulith** (horsegram) atta – by 6pm or as light dinner by itself or with rice	Make exercise a part of your daily life.
Acidity	BP Diabetes Indigestion Exhaustion PMS	Overnight soaked **raisins** – first thing in morning after waking up	**Dahi + soaked poha** – add salt + little green chilly – mid-meal	**Gulkand in water** – post dinner or sip through the day	Early bedtime and fixed wake up time.
Sweet cravings	Diabetes PCOd Kidney problems Vit b12/ Vit d deficiency Mood swings	Use of **Spices** in cooking – the way traditional recipes use them	**Roots and tuber vegetables** – like suran, arbi, etc- atleast 3-4 times a week	Add **peanut powder** to your meals – as chutney or on cooked salad (koshimbir)	Add ghee to all your main meals.
Tiredness/ lethargy	Thyroid PCOD Diabetes Low Hb Depression	**Aliv seeds** – as laddoo as mid meal or with milk at bedtime	Soaked **pulses** – sprouted and cooked – for lunch or dinner	Handful of **Cashews** – as a mid-meal – 11 am or 4 pm	Have seasonal sherbets

Urinary incontinence—loss of bladder control

Things you can do to prevent it and make a return to a healthy bladder

- Khareek (dry dates) first thing in morning.

- Sprouted and cooked moong and matki.
- One teaspoon of ghee with breakfast, lunch and dinner.
- Strength training and Kegel exercises.
- Yoga asanas (especially tadasana in Iyengar yoga method).

Afternoon nap

One who naps after lunch and walks after dinner never needs to see a physician—Arabic proverb.

Similar to the yogic concept of vamakukshi, nap post lunch when lying on the left side of the body, and shatapavali, a stroll of a hundred steps post dinner. The common thread of wisdom in different cultures is always based on common sense and is commonly forgotten.

Top five tips to rock the New Year party and feel spectacular the next day

1. Dal, rice or roti with paneer sabzi before leaving for the party. (A well-fed stomach comes with a brighter face and happier state of mind; basically ready to drink and dance the moment you arrive.)
2. Drink water between your drinks and eat peanuts, paneer, olives, fries, cheese—small stuff with good fats. (Stay well hydrated and don't let the alcohol hit you or drain you of your beauty or brains. Halka halka nasha chadhega.)
3. Eat something before you sleep—this is important. It could be khichdi, biryani or chivda or just bread and butter, but eat.
4. Wake up to a glass of water and eat some soaked raisins and one teaspoon of gulkand. (Nothing prevents

headaches or hangovers like this does, and also helps you cleanse your system.)
5. Eat a wholesome snack before noon. Moong dal chilla, or kulith pithala with bhakri, or boiled green grams (fresh ones) with kala namak, or egg and bread, or banana. (Essentially, take your pick but eat something.)

Alcohol

The only time that alcohol is healthy is when it is not consumed. But if you must drink it, here's what you can do:
1. Eat dinner before you drink.
2. Drink water between two drinks.
3. Don't drive when drunk.
4. Start the next day with a teaspoon of gulkand.
Issued in public interest.

The IPL diet

The players, broadcasters and owners are all making money, so why should we viewers get fat fukat mein.

Here's what you can do to stay fit while you watch the daily IPL game on TV:
1. Have chapatti with ghee and jaggery or ajwain paratha with white butter (makhan) or a banana by 6–6.30 p.m.
2. Khichdi-dahi or egg curry with rice or dal/sambar/fish with rice by 8.30–9 p.m.
3. Stand during the strategic time out, and between innings move to your window (Mumbai), or to your

veranda (rest of India) and stare into space. Allow the eyes and that brain some down time.
4. Stand and actually show what you mean every time you say, 'He should have played this shot like this.'
5. Drink milk or milk with gulkand or a protein shake before sleeping if you are the type that watches till the last ball and presentations.

Three food hacks that you can learn from Kareena Kapoor Khan

1. Start your day with a power-packed breakfast. If you have seen her killing it in the gym, know that her workout is being fuelled by kanda poha or aloo poha with dahi.
Tip: Eat that wholesome meal sixty to ninety minutes pre workout to ensure that you are able to optimise muscle fibre recruitment during exercise. This leads to a bigger afterburn (more calories burned post workout), and you get your results in a shorter period of time.
2. Nimbu pani with kala namak, sugar, kesar and a bit of ginger as a mid-afternoon pick-me-up drink (a couple of hours post lunch).
Tip: Keeps the afternoon slump away. The kesar works miracles for the hair and skin while the ginger and kala namak combo will leave you feeling light and helps avoid bloating on tough working days.
3. Dal-chawal-ghee or khichdi-dahi or doodhi sabzi and jowar roti with ghee for dinner.
Tip: An early and wholesome dinner ensures good, restorative sleep that helps the hormones stay in a state of

balance and has an anti-ageing effect on the body. Waking up fresh and sleeping soundly are the cornerstones of leading a good life.

Some tips for the hard-working corporate person

- If you are not waking up fresh in the mornings for over a month, it's probably because you need a break. Please take one ASAP.
- Ensure that you eat a meal on reaching office. If you find yourself having tea/coffee between 9 and 11 a.m. daily, it means that you are killing the hunger signal. Stop drinking and eat. Split breakfast into two meals. Have a small portion before leaving home and pack some for office.
- Keep a bottle of water on your table at all times and drink at least three bottles in office. Smoking (passive included), tea, coffee, and of course the air conditioners, make for a dehydrating environment.
- If you travel frequently, book flights which will let you have breakfast or dinner at home.
- If you haven't slept well or had a particularly stressful day, skip your workout and rest.
- Learn to help yourself. Cooking a few basic dishes such as dal-chawal, khichdi, chopping a salad for yourself doesn't just add to your sex appeal, it also makes tons of sense. It helps you unwind and reassures you that you do take care of your stomach and yourself.
- Never tell yourself that sleeping on the way to office and back while your driver is at the wheel makes up for the daily quota of sleep.

Travel tips

A life well-travelled is a life well lived. Some travel for fun, some for work, some to run away from the monotony of life, but irrespective of the reason, you do arrive. Arriving fresh is a bit of an art and therefore can be perfected with practice. A lot of my clients are passionate and ardent travellers, many even get photographed on arrival at the airports by the paparazzi. So here are the top eight secrets of travelling like you were born for it.

1. Eat a wholesome meal before you board the flight—irrespective of whether you are going home or away. Sandwich, rice and lentils, yoghurt and berries are a few good options, depending on where you are.
2. Drink up—but not the booze. Flights are dehydrating and the last thing you want to do is something that further dehydrates you. So not just booze, say no to the colas and packaged juices too.
3. Go slow—especially at the speed with which you chomp down your food. You are dehydrated and that is going to slow down your digestion. Eating less than usual but taking double the time to do so is the best way to prevent digestion problems. It takes time to learn to eat slow, but there's a flat stomach, smooth motions and glowing face at the end of it.
4. Walk—and ditch the escalators and lifts on landing. Not only will you win some envious stares, but your legs will thank you in the time to come. Sitting for long hours, whether in business, economy or yeah premium economy, is dreadful for the legs. A saggy lower body is a giveaway of age, so work it the minute you land.

5. Help your gut. Before you take a cab or train from the airport, pick up a yoghurt, kefir or home-set curd to revive the gut eco-system, lest the pressurised cabins or the travel stress gets to it. A natural source of vitamin B12, this will give you both the mental calm and the physical energy to find your way to the hotel/home post the journey.
6. Eat easy on reaching. Eat when you are at your destination, but spare a thought for the sluggish intestines. Fresh fruit, vegetables cooked with the right amount of spices and grains like rice and sorghum are easy to digest and will leave you feeling light.
7. Hot water bath—this is an Eastern hack for the world-weary. Not everyone can meditate, but everyone can have a bucket bath with hot water and crystals of salt. Ayurveda believes that salt belongs to the earth principle and can help one feel grounded. Especially recommended if you have a stressful meeting or a big deal to crack the next day.
8. Catch your routine wake-up time—don't sleep in. Regular travellers will vouch for the fact that jet lag is imaginary, the reality is that you are sleeping too much at the wrong time. So wake up, dust yourself off and learn to do surynamaskars. Just three rounds will be enough to open both your mind and the hips to explore and take in your travel and everything that comes with it.

Happy travels and know that you will get there with practice. May the wanderer in you live on forever.

Health tips for the frequent traveller

It looks glamorous from the outside but can take quite a toll on your health from the inside. Here are a few quick tips that help:

1. Travel

• Stay well hydrated. Carry a water bottle and keep sipping through the journey.

• Avoid chai and coffee on the flight and sixty minutes prior to boarding and post landing. (Okay for road trips though.)

2. Stay

• Pick hotels that offer gym access and yoga mats. If you travel to smaller places, buy a yoga mat, keep it in the hotel and ask for it every time you visit.

• Lie in supta baddha konasana for five minutes at bedtime.

3. Food

• Before you step out from your hotel, order khichdi/ dal-chawal/pasta for dinner and tell them what time they should send it to your room. If you wait to come back and order, you are calling for a pizza.

• Wherever possible, request for food from kitchen staff and not the restaurant, it's more like ghar ka khana.

• Carry peanuts, cashews, pistachios, etc. Chew on them between meetings and conferences and stay away from the pastries, cookies and biscuits.

Quarantine plan

Rujuta Diwekar

Here's a plan that will help you through the #lockdownextension. And while at it, will keep you strong, burn your fat and lift your mood.

Quarantine Plan 2.0

Note – The plan uses mostly non-perishables and some fresh fruits where available. Feel free to modify based on region, availability and taste. This plan is kid friendly.

Start your day

- Banana (constipation),
- Soaked almonds (diabetes, heart disease),
- Soaked raisins (PMS, Thyroid)

A healthy start sets the tone for the day. Puts you in the zone to balance chores at home and work from home.

Breakfast

- Poha, Upma, Idli, dosa, Paratha, egg & pav, etc.
- Deep fried wada or poori (once a week),
- Season special - mango milkshake

Homemade nashta helps keep your blood sugars and moods steady through the day.

Mid-Morning Snacks

- Nimbu, kokum or amla sherbets. OR a fresh fruit.

Lack of hydration leads to sugar cravings post lunch. Also, most sherbets and fruits are rich sources of Vit C which is a co-factor for iron assimilation and helps keep your Hb levels high.

Lunch

- Dal rice or roti sabzi + chutney (if you are low on micronutrients like B12 & D, also prevents afternoon slump)
- Banana & roti OR shikran poli (banana, sugar, milk and chapatti - if you are going through hot flushes or feeling gassy/ bloated)

Afternoon Snacks

- Dry coconut & jaggery or cashews & jaggery*
- Dry snacks like mathri, shankarpara, kurmura, chivda, chakli, etc.

*Mood enhancers, rich in essential fats and minerals, helps cut down on excesses of chai and coffee.

Workout

- 30 mins of workout daily
- 5 Suryanamaskar (good for all),
- Squats and lunges (for those struggling with a big paunch),
- Yoga practice (at your level, good for all)

Early Dinner

- Khichdi or dal/legumes with rice or phodni/ tadka/ vagharelo rice with an egg or paneer.

Easy to digest, cook and clean after. Legumes and rice are a good combo of essential and non-essential amino acids, fibre and protect the diversity and strength of good bacteria.

At Bedtime

- Haldi milk, the perfect night cap, improves sleep quality and that protects the immune system.
- Add nutmeg, if you suffer from insomnia or weak digestion.
- Add dry ginger, for weak bones, joints, low strength.
- Add 1-2 strands of kesar for better skin and hair.

Good Habits

- Nap in the afternoon, not more than 20 - 30 mins.
- Regulate gadget use. Keep the phone at a fixed place at home. It's a strategy that will cut down usage by at least 30 mins a day.
- Sit down for at least one meal a day, chew slowly, eat silently.
- Be in your own company, it's not as scary as you think it.

Section Four

FOOD IS FOR EVERYONE

“

RUJUTA SAYS...

Exercise is the best drug you can be on. Good looks is the only side effect.

The tendency of the body is to be lazy and that of the mind to be wavering. So, inspired by nature, yoga was developed as a practice to help the body move and keep the mind still.

People who exercise should care about how light they feel on their feet and not on the scales.

You can't escape pain but you can choose where to have it. The fit have it in their muscles and the un-fit in their joints.

Exercise is the seat belt you need to wear to prevent any diet accidents in your life journey.

Very simply, the best exercise is the one that gets done on a regular basis.

”

4A. EXERCISE AND YOGA

A well-fuelled system is naturally active. It allows you to take the stairs instead of the lift, use public transport (or a bike) instead of the car, and stand instead of sit. Essentially, it keeps the body the way it was meant to be: full of movement.

Exercise is the ultimate happiness drug that you could ever lay your hands on; it actually puts the brain into a euphoric state without the dangers of hitting a low later on. To repeat a wise saying i once heard: there are bad days, and then there are days when you exercise.

How much to exercise

Most of us feel fat now, or have felt so for fifteen years or more. But when you log into Facebook today, a picture of yours from two, five or seven years ago crops up. Suddenly, you realise that you look thin in 'memories'. So, you know that your current look might appear to be 'very thin' to you two years from now.

Essentially, this means two things. 1. You are constantly feeling fat. 2. Whatever you are doing today is progressively making you fat for the years to come. Here's a simple way to reverse that.

Get rid of the weighing scale and get yourself an exercise calendar instead. You know this but it's worth repeating—weight is a useless thing to lose. Body weight is not an indicator of our fatness or fitness; it is compliance to exercise that indicates fitness. Research in the field of exercise science says that exercising is four times more effective than losing weight when it comes to good health and protection from lifestyle diseases like diabetes, heart health, etc. These are the kind of reports that we should be reading, but they never make it to the media. From the brain to the gut, from insulin to adipose tissue, from the bones to the nerves, exercise is uplifting and should be a non-negotiable aspect of our lives.

We also now know that we don't need to kill ourselves in the gym; instead, we need only 150 minutes of exercise a week to see changes in our body composition—'weight loss' to the uninitiated. That's all it takes to keep every lifestyle disease, including obesity, at bay. Weekly 150 minutes accommodates for rough times at work, holidays, guests, bad weather, bad mood, basically for life in general.

The next time you look at a picture from your past, don't think of how much weight you have gained but how many hours of exercise you have lost.

Work out as you will

Swimming is the best exercise. No, wait, walking is. Hmm, how about yoga? That's good and safe for everyone, right? So what's the official word on that?

Just like there's no 'right man/ideal woman' to get married to, it changes in each phase of our life, there is no 'best' exercise. But unlike relationships, with exercise, you have the option of moving from one to another without a sense of guilt or betrayal. The 'best' exercise is one that engages you physically, mentally, emotionally, and on levels even deeper than that. It is something that you look forward to on a daily basis, it is the reason you eat dinner on time, it is the reason you hit the bed early. It is the reason you wake up even before your alarm goes off.

It makes you feel beautiful inside out, it keeps you young, makes you smile, fall in love with yourself all over again. Yes, the 'right' exercise has that magical effect on all of us, it can calm our nerves, sharpen our memory, erase those worry lines, flatten that bulge under the eye and over the stomach and make you light and contented like a happy child.

It is up to us to seek the 'right' exercise, because there are no set rules on how to keep the body in top shape. Information so authoritatively dispensed by various tabloids and social media influencers, or at a bout of party gossip, can't rule our heads or heart when it comes to making decisions about our workout. Some of us will find it in yoga, some of us in running, some find it in pumping iron and others while biking at dawn. The question is, are you searching?

Right foot forward

'Sweat it out,' we are told, burn some fat. True lies. In a hot country like ours, we can all sweat it out even while waiting for a bus or waiting for the valet to bring the car. But does that lead to a smaller waist, a six-pack or accelerated fat burning? No, it simply means smelly bodies.

The point i am making is that exercise is a non-negotiable aspect of our lives, but 'sweating it out' should be understood as a metaphor for it, and not taken literally. Chase fitness, not sweat.

Working out has three main subjects—flexibility, strength and cardio-respiratory fitness.

Way too often, we bother only about the cardio-respiratory fitness part. Doctors tell us to 'go take a walk'. Obediently, we walk and walk and walk, and come back with sprained ankles, bad backs and weak knees.

What we don't realise is that walking, which is supposed to be great for the heart, can be detrimental to tendons, ligaments and joints if you get fanatical about it. To walk effectively, without damaging your body, you need to make time for resistance training to build strength and stretching to build flexibility. You can use your body weight or dumbbells or bars or gym equipment for resistance training. A qualified professional will help you figure out what is the right resistance exercise for you. Stretching, as part of a warm-up for exercise and as a cool-down after exercise, helps make the joints flexible. Yoga asanas, learnt from an experienced teacher, will help build all-round fitness, though with much less sweat than the other options.

The bottom line: Seek professional guidance, spend time and money to work out an exercise schedule that will improve your overall fitness. Never adopt somebody else's regime, or the most popular one of the moment—it could do you more harm than good.

Don't just sit around

'i have no time to exercise, can i still lose weight?' Ah! By now you already know that it's not about losing weight, it's about getting fit and improving your body composition: more lean mass, less fat mass ... So the short answer to the above question is NO.

Unless you invest time in exercising, as well as eating right, fitness will just be ... a living-room conversation topic for you. But don't lose hope if you don't have time to exercise (which i don't believe); the one thing you can do while you're struggling to get that exercise routine going is cut down on the amount of time you spend sitting.

Sitting down for more than thirty minutes at a time is fast-emerging as the single biggest factor influencing metabolic syndrome, the condition linked to a host of obesity-related diseases. Our lifestyles today are full of sitting down—to work, to eat, to watch TV, to have coffee, to travel on flights, to talk things out, on a romantic date ... sit, sit, sit—we seem to do nothing else. And the longer we sit, the bigger our medical bills. That's because sitting is changing not just the size of our pants, it's also making many invisible changes in our bodies, including our intracellular environment. Our hormones and enzymes seem to be at a loss about how to come to terms with how much time we spend sitting. And the webinars are not helping.

The biggest toll that sitting around takes is on insulin sensitivity. The insulin in our bodies is finding it tougher to transport nutrients and glucose to cells without the support of bodily movement. Blood sugar stays high, the cells starve, the insulin feels overworked, the body cries out for help—and we keep sitting. So watch that clock, get up and walk around before the thirty minutes are up. And sign up for that gym class, now.

Workout or diet?

Workout or diet, what is more effective? Choosing between the two is like choosing between two loved ones or between the devil and the deep blue sea, depending on your outlook. Both complement each other and any diet programme that doesn't promote exercise (not just walking) is not going to improve your metabolic parameters or reduce risk to diseases.

An effective diet is one that improves the efficiency of your workout and lets you do more with your body—wake up earlier, run faster, lift stronger, stay longer in an asana, work later in the night, etc. Being low on energy and needing a coffee/tea to get through a meeting is the first sign that you will not go to the gym or that yoga class, and that even if you really push yourself to get there, you will break more than build fitness.

An effective workout is one that promotes sensible eating, not the one that is so 'effective' that you can eat anything and still lose weight. A good workout is one that follows the main principle of exercise—progressive overload—and teaches your body to do more and not less with age. Doing more with the body is so uplifting that it motivates you to not eat the pastry, not party till late and not put the alarm on snooze.

Anyway, i know what you meant by effective, the one that lets you drop weight on the scales. But then, health, wellness and fitness could never be measured by a number. So, if you really want an effective weight-loss plan, get off the scales and worry about how you feel, not whether you fit into that dress.

A quick lesson in exercise physiology (Yu kasrat karte karte, kaahe ko hum mare?)

Too often we have been told to reduce weight be it to look better, lower diabetes, BP or simply to get married.

But we have been told the wrong stuff.

If you really want to look better, have well controlled blood sugar and BP levels, then what you should be doing is working on improving your strength to weight ratio. Essentially you should gear your training and eating in a way that allows your muscles to hypertrophy (become big) and bones to become dense (heavy). When this happens, in lay terms we call it a toned body. A toned body means that you look slim but not sick.

Losing weight and the methods people employ to do it—crash diets, detox farms, 'fasting', excessive exercise that includes mainly cardio, etc.—often leads to the exact opposite, i.e., loss of bone mineral density and muscle tissue. You could now weigh less but look flabbier in the same or even smaller size clothes.

To cut a long story short, if you are fuming in the gym, you will be smiling outside it. Train hard, stay strong, shut that weight-loss machine in your head.

Recruit those muscle fibres

Exercise is all about muscle fibre recruitment (MFR). More the number of muscle fibres you put to work, higher fat burning is what you get. E.g., squats recruit more muscle fibres than crunches.

Factors influencing MFR:

- Choice of exercise—strength training recruits max muscle fibres.
- Duration—not more than sixty minutes.
- Sequence—work the big muscles before small muscles.
- Frequency—overtraining and ignoring rest compromises on MFR and exposes you to injury.

Why you must squat

The full squat! Once upon a time, the preferred Indian pose to detox. Be it in the loo or in the chowrasta to gossip away with friends and neighbours.

In training terms, it's a good test for the strength and flexibility in your lower body.

It also:

- Builds bone density.
- Prevents thighs from bulging out from the sides of your jeans.
- Helps beat PMS mood swings and menstrual cramps.
- Improves insulin sensitivity and helps you beat diabetes, PCOD and obesity.
- Boosts sleep quality.
- Ensures that you don't crack under pressure in real life.

In pursuit of a flat stomach—deadlifts

Alright, so a flat stomach is always elusive. Not so much because you are carrying excess fat but because you are carrying too little strength.

Strength is amongst the least celebrated aspects of fitness, but is in fact the key to low fat mass, improved bone density, hormonal balance, etc.

The deadlift is the baap of all exercises, and yet amongst the most misunderstood ones.

It's as dangerous as crossing the road, driving a car or talking to your boss about a sticky matter. It's all about technique. It's about how you do it and knowing when to stop. i would put it in the low-risk, high-reward category.

Every girl must learn to lift at least the equivalent of her body weight. So if you are 60 kg, you should be able to lift at least 60 kg. That's what you should train for, aspire for, eat for.

Chalo, lift.

All about exercise

Part 1

Our lifespans are increasing and our health is deteriorating. Exercise bridges this gap and enables us to lead a better quality of life.

Beyond the obvious benefits, this is what exercise does to our BBHH.

Brain:

• Leads to better neural network, prevents Alzheimer's, dementia, forgetfulness, etc.

• Improves neurogenesis in dentate gyrus, the learning centre in the brain.
• Fights depression and improves confidence.

Bones:

• Allows bones and joints to assimilate minerals like calcium. Without the stimuli of exercise, calcium from food or supplements cannot be assimilated properly.
• Increases bone mineral density and prevents osteoporosis.

Heart:

• Increases the capillary network in the left ventricle (LV), making the heart much more efficient.
• Makes the heart muscle stronger/bigger.
• Reduces resting heart rate.
• Controls blood pressure.

Hormones:

• Improves insulin sensitivity and helps beat diabetes.
• Regulates the growth hormone for better skin and hair.
• Regulates cortisol for better quality sleep in the night and alertness in the day.

Part 2

In Part 1, we learned that exercise is not just important, but critical for a good quality of life. But for exercise to be effective, it has to be in a proper structure.

The most important principles which help you plan and structure your exercise program:

Progressive overload—Exercise volume and intensity need to increase progressively over a period of time. Without this, it is no longer an exercise but becomes an activity. For example, over a period of time, a run/walk should either cover more distance in the same time or become longer in duration.

Adaptation—Takes place in response to the progressive overload. Our body adapts by getting stronger/fitter in response to the exercise stimuli. Nutrition and hydration are critical to the recovery processes that allow for the adaptation response to set in.

RPE—And how do you decide if your body has adapted? By using the RPE scale. Rate of perceived exertion measures your effort levels on a scale of one to ten. Any exercise which starts at level eight, for example, will soon become six or lower, and this means adaptation has happened and the exercise dose needs to be increased so that RPE becomes eight again.

Part 3

Just like diets, exercise needs to be sustainable for it to be a success. Most of us are guilty of either doing too much or too little and most times nothing. So here's a sample weekly exercise chart that can be followed. You can modify it depending on your current exercise routine.

Important rules for exercise planning:

- Keep a two-day gap at least between two weight-training sessions.
- Schedule cardio a day after weight training.
- Build in recovery days to get the best out of exercise days.
- Yoga asanas are an excellent form of exercise, recovery and much more. (And can be done daily.)
- Plan for at least 150 minutes of total workout time in the week.

Weekly exercise calendar:
Day 1: Weight training
Day 2: Forty minutes of cardio—easy run/swim/cycling/dance
Day 3: Active rest/yoga asana
Day 4: Weight training
Day 5: Yoga asana/hobby
Day 6: Twenty minutes speed workout—sprints/jumps, etc.
Day 7: Active rest (stay active, move around).

Part 4

What you eat is the most undervalued but crucial aspect of making exercise work for you. Here are the top five foods that improve exercise performance:

1. Rice: Easy to digest, rice is a prebiotic (food for probiotic bacteria) and a good source of BCAA (branch chain amino acids). Especially important for people who are into intense exercises as the RS3 (a specific type of starch found in rice) helps keep the gut strong and enhances exercise performance. Choose the local, hand-pounded or single-polished variety and not brown rice.
2. Aliv or garden cress seeds: Rich in folic acid and iron, this one is best absorbed after being soaked in coconut water and rolled into a laddoo with coconut and jaggery. Alternatively, have the soaked aliv seeds post a meal or mix them in milk for a nightcap (details in *Indian Superfoods*).
3. Coconut: God's own food for keeping the immunity and fat-burning processes strong. Best consumed in all the familiar ways—tender, ripe, dry and not to forget the

ALL ABOUT EXERCISE

It's not just important but crucial that we exercise

WHY? ABUNDANCE OF BENEFITS...

BRAIN
- **Prevents** Forgetfulness, Alzheimer, Dementia etc.
- **Fights** Depression
- **Improves** Neurogenesis in dentate gyrus, the learning centre in the brain

BONES
- **Assimilates** Calcium
- **Improves** bone mineral density
- **Prevents** Osteoporosis

HEART
- **Strengthens** Heart muscles
- **Reduces** Resting heart rate
- **Controls** Blood pressure

HORMONES
- **Improves** Insulin sensitivity and helps beat diabetes
- **Regulates** growth hormone (GH) for better skin and hair
- **Regulates** Cortisol for better quality sleep in the night and alertness in the day

HOW? BY FOLLOWING A PROPER STRUCTURE

RULES FOR EXERCISE PLANNING

- Keep atleast a 2 day gap between two weight training sessions
- Schedule cardio a day after weight training
- Build in recovery days to get the best out of exercise days
- Yoga asanas are an excellent form of exercise, recovery and much more (And can be done daily)
- Plan for at least 150 mins of total workout time in the week

WEEKLY EXERCISE CALENDAR*

* You can modify depending on your current exercise routine

DAY 1	DAY 2	DAY 3	DAY 4	DAY 5	DAY 6	DAY 7
Weight training	40 CARDIO Easy run/ swim/ cycling/ dance	Active rest/ Yoga asana	Weight training	Yoga asana/ Hobby	20 SPEED WORKOUTS Sprints/ jumps, etc.	Active rest

WHAT TO EAT? EATING RIGHT IS CRUCIAL TO ENSURE THAT EXERCISE WORKS FOR YOU

Pre-workout meal

Have a fruit 15-20 mins before a workout or a main meal 60-90 mins before

4 R's of Post workout meal

- **Rehydrate** Drink enough water to quench your thirst and then have some more
- **Replenish** Replenish the glycogen stores with a fruit like banana
- **Repair** Drink a whey protein shake to help in the repair processes
- **Recover** Have anti-oxidants like Vit C, Vit E, Selenium, Zinc, etc., for quick recovery

Zinc Vitamin C Vitamin E Selenium

TOP 5 FOODS TO IMPROVE EXERCISE PERFORMANCE

RICE — Hand pounded; Keeps the gut strong; Easy to digest; Local; Prebiotic; Single polished; Avoid brown rice; Good source of BCAA

TUBERS — Sabudana; Arbi; Rich in fibre; Good for women; Rich in minerals; Sweet potato; Suran; Rich in vitamins; Keeps our hormones balanced; For skin glow

ALIV — Indian superfood; Garden Cress Seeds; Rich in folic acid; Rich in iron

WHEY PROTEIN — Right ratio of essential to non essential amino acids; Useful for the older adults who are exercising routinely; Easy on the stomach; Speed up your recovery

COCONUT — Consume tender, ripe, dry and the water; Regulates blood pressure; Strong immunity

Rujuta Diwekar

water (regulates blood pressure also). Have it as part of a wholesome meal and avoid the new fads like adding it to coffee, etc.

4. Tubers like sweet potato, suran, arbi and even sabudana (tapioca/cassava): Especially good for women in fitness as, along with the fibre, vitamins and minerals, these work at keeping our hormones in a state of balance. Want skin that keeps the exercise glow for a long time? These forgotten veggies could well be your secret route to that.

5. Whey protein: First amongst equals in the world of supplements, especially useful for older adults who are exercising routinely. A fine balance of essential to non-essential amino acids that is easy on the stomach. Make it a part of your post-workout routine and speed up your recovery (details in *Don't Lose Out, Work Out!*).

THE BHARATNATYAM BUTT

As a daughter of a middle-class Maharashtrian family, along with school i was also enrolled in a classical dance class. Thankfully for me, i loved it and my teacher was least interested in pushing her kids to take exams. That way we had endless time to sit in aramandi (the half-squat posture), practice adavaus (basic steps or alphabets of dancing) and learn hastas (hand mudras or positions). As i grew up, i realised that many people feel that Bharatnatyam gives you a largish appearance and a big butt. The truth is that all it gives you, other than the ability to appreciate art in all forms, is a strong spine, well-formed gluteus (hips) and well-balanced hormones.

i am thirty-eight and i must have started my periods may be when i was fifteen, and in so many years my back hasn't even hurt once. So at least twenty-three years x twelve periods and it doesn't hurt, cramp, ache even once. And instead of focusing on the benefits, all that gets talked about is Bharatnatyam and the hip size! Are my hips big? Yes, but only compared to my waist, and i am more than cool with it.

Coz as i look back, i know that it's exposure to classical art early in life that allows for delayed puberty when young and a sense of comfort with the body as we get old.

Running

It reminds you of the freedom in your joints and a mind that you enjoyed as a child. It makes you a believer in car-free roads, it teaches you that you don't necessarily have to stop to smell the roses, it makes you come alive with the spirit that you had long-forgotten but still dwells within you.

Train, then run for your life

Another marathon, another flood of injuries, another round of warnings from medical professionals about running being bad for the knees and another year of training in the exact same way. Mumbai, Delhi, Bangalore—it's the same story. There is no denying that running is a favoured activity of the urban Indian. i can add 'middle-aged' to that. If you are not part of a running group, you are not cool. Peer pressure, lifestyle guilt, need for a social life—and for a small minority, the love for running. Whatever your reason, now that you have decided to run, do justice to your choice.

There are two things you need to focus on to make sure you are not just a participator and to avoid injuries—strengthening and stretching. Running puts unprecedented mechanical force on your tendons, bones, ligaments and joints (TBLJ), the weak points in your body; much weaker than the heart and lungs. Weight training in the gym lets you strengthen and lubricate your joints, adds to your bone mineral density and yes, increases the capillary network in your heart, making it a stronger muscle. Make sure you follow the right technique and build up the intensity gradually.

Stretching before and after the run is a concept we all understand but often overlook. It gets the blood flow to the muscles involved in running and prepares them for their full range of motion. During training, stretching is as crucial as the run itself. Make sure you dedicate enough time and thought to that.

Change the way you train, and remember, it's not running that leads to injuries, it's only running.

Guidelines for marathon runners

Before the run

- Take it easy, it's time to slow down not just training but even the way you chew food. Slower = better digestion = better glycogen stores.

• Cut down on excesses—tea, coffee, alcohol. Anything that dehydrates comes in the way of good performance.
• Plan your breakfast (no packaged cereals) and 6 p.m. meal (wholesome) in advance and eat rice for dinner.
• Homemade dahi and chaas with ajwain, jeera, for your gut health.
• No new foods this week.

During the run

• Start the day with a banana/local fruit.
• Carry soaked raisins for the run—it's easier on the stomach.
• Don't try gels if you haven't practised that in training.
• Walk when you sip water.

Post the run

• Keep sipping on water.
• Boiled potato and white bread sandwich after the run. Quick and easy to digest.
• Khichdi and dahi for lunch.
• Homemade fried food in the evening to ensure that there is no calorie deficit or loss of immunity.
• Make time to stretch twice before you go to bed.
• Good sleep and a light twenty-minute workout the next day.
• No alcohol for seventy-two hours post the run.

Sprinting uphill

• Improves fat burning over the next forty-eight hours.
• Maximum recruitment of the core.
• Quickest route to reducing girth.
• Lowers resting heart rate and BP.
• Helps regulate blood sugars naturally.

Yoga

A beginner's guide to yoga

The yoga tradition is more than 5,000 years old and it is orally documented and passed on through the guru–shishya parampara or lineage. The wisdom of yoga is more subjective than objective. Yoga gurus would carefully handpick competent students and groom them to become acharyas or teachers.

Recently, i met a man, ninety-two years young, who asked me about the benefits of yoga, only to reveal that his enthusiasm, energy and youth came out of his consistent practice of sarvangasana for five minutes every day for the entire length of his life. This breed of men and women who practice for a few minutes but as a part of daily discipline is becoming rare. Yoga is now practised more for perceived benefits than just as a matter of daily discipline.

And a lot of this is because yoga is now no longer just an art and science but a full-fledged industry. This doesn't take away from the art itself but makes it quite a challenge to choose the right yoga class.

Here are some quick tips:

Yoga, like love ...

- ... is right for you the day it happens. So age, gender, nationality, race, religion, etc., don't matter.
- ... doesn't expect you to give up on your own life, instead becomes an integral part of yours.
- ... doesn't grudge you for having a social life or work commitments, instead makes it easier to maintain that elusive work-life balance.

Yoga basics:

• Yoga is learnt in class but 'done' outside when you practice the equanimity it teaches. Yoga is beyond asana or physical postures.

• It teaches you that the body must be used as a learning tool so that life can be more fulfilling on every front—career, family, hobby, etc.

• Believes that as the body changes, the practice should adapt so that optimum health and fitness can be enjoyed forever.

• Doesn't believe in 'sweating it out', rather it takes a more nurturing approach, a disciplined one nevertheless.

Yoga in practice:

• Keeps your body lean, toned and light.

• Works on strength, stamina, stability and flexibility in every asana.

• Teaches you to hold one part of the body, and to let go of another.

• Choose a class based on the teacher and not on the promise of weight loss or nirvana.

Yoga teacher:

• Should have a solid base of daily asana practice. Focused on learning and not just earning.

• Should encourage you to challenge your body's limits every time but in a safe, effective and non-pushy manner.

• Takes the effort to acquaint you with the Sanskrit names of the asanas and doesn't refer to adhomukhasvanana as dog pose for years together.

• Promotes a holistic, sustainable way of life, one that is away from fads. Including the yoga industry fads.

Yoga business:

• Like it or not, yoga is now a BIG industry. Just the million-dollar apparel and yoga mat business went up by another 50 per cent in the last four years.

• The chances of you running into a yoga business model is always higher than you running into a yoga school.

• But much like love, once you find true yoga, it's a life-changing experience.

On meditation

'An agitated mind cannot meditate.' When i read that in *Light on Life* by B.K.S. Iyengar, it struck me like a bolt of lightning. The internet is loaded with information about meditation and how to quickly get there with scents, chants and some yoga poses. The by-lanes of Rishikesh, the yoga capital of the world, are filled with banners and posters of programs that teach you to meditate in as little as three days with a certificate to boot. All this and still meditation remains a mystery.

Of the eight steps of Ashtanga yoga, as Patanjali laid it out, meditation or dhyana is the seventh step, just before samadhi or complete nirvana. Unlike what is commonly understood, it's a state that one arrives at after years of practice, the practice of leading a disciplined life, one that teaches us at the very least to eat, sleep and talk in moderation.

Honestly, i am not even sure if there is a guide to meditation or if i can write one, but i will surely tell you what i have heard from various yoga masters about this ancient spiritual practice. This may strike you as pretty basic or simple, but then we all know one thing, simplicity is profound.

These are the steps that the yoga masters have laid out:

- Wake and sleep at a fixed hour every day.
- Wake up before the sun rises and watch how the morning arrives to the sound of the singing birds and swaying branches around you.
- Adopt an exercise routine that you stick to daily.
- Suryanamaskar is especially beneficial as it brings a rhythm to both the body and the breath.
- Eat food that is cooked and served with love.
- Maintain silence around mealtimes and be grateful for what's on your plate.
- Make food choices that lead to heeta or wellbeing of all living beings on earth.
- Build a bedtime routine that allows you to unwind.
- Stay off gadgets at least an hour before sleep and spend some time in silence, just with yourself, before you hit the bed.
- Begin and end your day with a prayer.
- Meditation in photographs is different from what it is in reality; be prepared to recognise the difference when you practice it in real life.
- The path is beautiful if you take it a step at a time.
- The journey is the destination of meditation.

The right eats for yoga

'But they say you should do yoga on an empty stomach!' This is what i often hear from my clients and on my Facebook page. So often that i have stopped wondering why 'they' don't mention 'yama' and 'niyama', the two crucial aspects of Patanjali Yoga Sutras that precede asana and pranayama. Yama and niyama can be loosely translated as restraints and observances that one must follow to make the most of one's life or at least to derive maximum benefits out of asana and pranayama practice. They aren't esoteric but rather common sense 'laws' which can improve one's physical, mental and emotional wellbeing.

One such yama is mitahar, the ability to eat the right food at the right time, pretty much aligning itself to the 'everything in moderation' wisdom. Though there is no direct reference in yogic scriptures to 'don't eating anything' in the morning before practice, there are many references to overeating and even a warning that one must not overeat: 'A light stomach aids asana and pranayama practice'.

Now, we modern yogis have reduced or 'adapted' this to 'do yoga on an empty stomach in the morning'. Conveniently forgetting that a light stomach is attained by early dinners, regular bedtimes, good bowel movements—an entire lifestyle. This isn't instant noodles where all that matters is what you ate two minutes before starting your asana or pranayama. Late-night binges or that fancy restaurant dinner after which you crashed in the car all lead to a dull and clogged gastro-intestinal tract—not conducive to asana practice and completely out of tune with yama or niyama.

So my dear yogi, wake up and smell the coffee (not literally). Early dinners—that should be thy focus. A fruit in the morning will not make your system 'heavy', late dinners will.

Top four points from my talk at The International Yoga Conference in Beijing

1. Anna he purna Brahma. Every grain of food we eat is a representation of the eternal truth. Eat like you're praying; food is a blessing not some random number of calories.
2. Knowing when to stop eating is the sign of highest wisdom (*Hatha Yoga Pradipika*). To eat according to one's need, and not greed, is to eat in awareness, and is called mitahar, one of the yamas of yoga philosophy.
3. To eat satvic is to eat food that is simple, sensible and seasonal. The reason why yoga has gone global is because it teaches practicality and responsibility as the stepping stone to spirituality. It encourages us to eat right without being fussy or obsessive about food.
4. Sukhasana, silence and sharing—the three fundamentals to prepare the mind for meditation. Anna and mana, food and its influence on the mind, was studied deeply by the yogis. Eating while maintaining a simple cross-legged posture and silence, along with the ability to share from your plate, were simple but effective steps towards teaching the mind the discipline required to progress in yoga practice.

Food for yoga practitioners

If you are a yoga practitioner, then you are a no-nonsense person. The type that practices asanas more than poses for it. Not in fear of the deadly virus but cautious anyway.

As the world goes through an unprecedented lockdown, the attention has come back to food, especially foods for immunity. So are there foods that can help keep the joints mobile, mind free and body immune? Yes, there are. From the traditional wisdom of Indian kitchens and the shastras of Ayurveda and yoga. Here goes a quick list:

• Ginger in all forms. For once, adrak chai is just what the doctor prescribed. Traditionally used to spice up life, beat flus and coughs and to improve bones and joints, the ginger can truly uplift your spirits in dull times. Add it to your soups, grate it over your baked beans or simply have it with your cup of chai.

• Haldi or turmeric. Flavour of the season in the West, but the herb that has stood the test of time in India. From being used as an external application on the bride before the day of the wedding, to being used in the daily cooking of dals, to simply being added to milk and turned into a nightcap, haldi is amongst the most versatile of all spices. An immunity booster, antioxidant and what have you. Special tip: Mix equal amounts of ghee, turmeric and ginger, roll into nail-sized balls and have it post practice or at bedtime.

• Til or sesame. Rich in vitamins and essential fats, til is known for everything from boosting immunity to improving skin and bone health. You can roast a few seeds and add it to steamed veggies for lunch, you can have tahini over a crispy toast for breakfast or cook a nice khichdi for dinner in til oil.

• Amla or the Indian gooseberry. Rich in vitamin C and bioactive agents that prevent free radical damage, improve immune function and boost respiratory health. As chyawanprash, a traditional preparation using amla, ghee and spices, as pickle or simply drying amla to turn it into a salty or sweet candy, it's good for you in all forms. Especially useful for senior practitioners.

• Khichdi. Any combination of the humble pulses like moong or toor and rice is India's most open secret of a pick-me-up or a light meal. At once it's a meal that prevents illnesses and even aids recovery from them. A combination that is light on the stomach, also works as prebiotic (food for good bacteria) and helps in assimilation of nutrients and expulsion of toxins from the body.

• Other secrets from the Indian kitchens include kulith or horse gram, a pulse that boosts energy and makes for a source of veg protein. And ragi or finger millet—a treasure trove of antioxidants and minerals, which prevent illness and ensures that the body has a robust immune response. Quick reminder: Guruji B.K.S. Iyengar often said that the best way to boost the immune function is to practice.

A guru in the age of experts

Tea, he declared, slapping his hands on his knees as he got up from the chair. i followed him first to the kitchen and then to the garden which faced the Bhagirathi. Swami Govindananda settled on the bench. i sat much ahead of him on the green grass, staring at the river and the huge green mountain across, and at the women working in the fields nearby.

'i can watch this scene for the rest of my life sitting here,' i declared to him. 'No,' he said in his south Indian accent, 'you will get bored.' 'Yeda ho gaya hai kya?' i said to him, non-verbally of course. He heard it. 'Boredom, lethargy is natural to the mind. Right now, it's new, so it's stimulating, even entertaining, then you will get bored.' Beyond a point, i don't talk even in my head so i said nothing. But Swamiji was always philosophical without meaning to be so.

It was a month-long course and he was our resident teacher, a teacher to twenty-five, thirty students from across the globe studying yoga at this remote ashram near Uttarkashi. He was, in fact, the designated swami for the Sivananda tradition to be deputed whenever they were starting a project/ashram in any remote location. He could get all things and people moving—a rare mix of physical vigour and mental calm.

During those thirty days, he gave me enough chaabi to trek alone. That i was line-maroing Stefan (full story in *Land of Moonlit Snows*) didn't bother him. He was not the typical teacher, reminding me of what i was here for, surely not for ishq-vishq, or the typical middle-aged man, who gets all protective and says but what's the future with this guy? The thing is that he was and very much is, an embodiment of all that yoga and Ayurveda teach. Mostly, he has the bandwidth to practice what he teaches, effortlessly, in real life. He isn't scared of the workings of daily life, youth or even hormones, and he has the unshakable confidence that his students will walk the right path even when they don't seem to in that moment.

Recently there was a blog on a hundred yoga gurus of India, and i was thrilled to see the names of many people i know on the list. Swamiji featured on it too and i wondered what he thought about it. If there's a list, it's not yoga, he may say.

i feel in a world where yoga has been so commercialised, teachers like him who follow the path like it was meant to be—live, eat, learn with students—are a rare commodity. Of course, there's the teaching of classical yoga texts, but beyond that, there is no Sanskrit verse that he throws at you. Instead, he picks his own plate after eating, washes his own cup after chai, picks the broom to clean the yoga hall. No vulnerabilities to be capitalised on and no cultivation of followers. Access is free, 24/7 and unconditional. In yoga, the teaching is important, not the teacher, he would say.

To all the gurus of classical forms, be it yoga, Ayurveda, dance or music, for all those who stay true to traditions of empowerment in the age of social media followers, tweetable quotes and Instagrammable posts, happy Guru Purnima. May your tribe increase.

Hari Om Tat Sat, Swamiji.

An ode to Guruji B.K.S. Iyengar

'i teach sensible, not sensual, yoga,' roared the ninety-four-year-old yoga guru to a mesmerised crowd of over 1,200 students in Guangzhou, China, in 2011.

If they were not in trikonasana at the time—lifting the sides of the waist and extending their arms from their 'armpit chest'—they would have applauded. This was the first time that the trikonasana felt like a proper triangle, the body felt united by being divided in multiple triangles.

It was for the first time they felt an uninterrupted flow of energy from the bone to muscle, from muscle to the skin and from the skin back to the bones.

It was the first time that Bellur Krishnamachar Sundararaja Iyengar himself was in that country, stimulating and satiating the Chinese hunger for yoga. It was amazing to see this yoga artiste overcome the language barrier to teach each one of us when in his nineties—his enthusiasm and energy could put a nine-year-old to shame. It was like he had an eye on each one of us; it was a surreal experience.

Though not even a shadow of the master's greatness, skill, expertise, knowledge and wisdom, i too was invited for the same Sino–India health and yoga summit for a small talk on the food wisdom that yoga offers. That's how i happened to be there.

The reason why i made it at thirty-four to China to teach or speak about food wisdom is because, for eighty-seven years of his life, Guruji had walked the path of fire and taught yoga to people who were not even interested in learning. He was an inspiration.

During an interview earlier that year, he had told me that people in Pune, where he had been sent by his guru T. Krishnamachari, were so upset by his endeavours to teach yoga that they resorted to black magic, not just to rid him from Pune, but the country itself of yoga. i feel part of that black magic worked, because Iyengar and his methodology of yoga transcended not just the boundaries of Pune, but the entire country.

Interest in the West was kindled by Guruji's approach, and it was stoked constantly with his logical, technical and yet sensitive approach to yoga. It was exactly what the world was waiting for. Technology of the West, culture of the East. Brain of the West, heart of the East. He did it by applying physiological and anatomical understanding to an art that was purely orally transmitted. He refined it by using terms that were physiologically correct but easily understood.

He taught yoga not because he was keen to tell you what he knows, but keen to learn how to apply his art to everybody. Iyengar was put to test multiple times. He would mostly get students that every doctor or medical science had rejected as a hopeless case; they would not just recover completely but many of them are currently teachers themselves.

The easiest thing would have been to mystify what he does with each one of them, say that this sequence of asanas or the aids—be it the use of bricks, belts, bolsters, bench, blankets—that he used to help them overcome their shortcomings, a stiff back/neck/hamstring, broken bones or malignant tumours, etc., came to him in meditation or some such exotic thing. Instead, he went out of his way to demystify, to explain how it worked physiologically, how certain asanas could make it easier for the ovaries to receive blood supply, or the heart to reduce its diastolic pressure, for example.

He made sure that no one saw him as a man of God, but as a man of discipline. It is because of his work that people today are interested in the Eastern sciences. It is because people, after their long exposure to Iyengar's work, know that it is not some rope trick humbug, it is real science. That is exactly what a yoga guru does—paves the way for an uninterrupted flow of intelligence to reach the next generation, even if the present generation doesn't possess adequate skills to transmit or understand it in totality.

Like the sage Patanjali, the founding father of yoga, Iyengar possessed not just an intuitive understanding of Ayurveda and the workings of the body, but also the gift of using words in a powerful and imaginative manner. Like Patanjali's skill over grammar, Iyengar developed an almost new vocabulary that made it easy for students across the globe to understand exactly how their bodies are meant to move, to experience and perform a certain asana in its purest form.

Extending from the 'armpit chest' or moving the 'dorsal spine' in, gets even a lay person with no background of physiology, anatomy, etc., to understand the working of the human body. It allows them to understand and employ the voluntary muscles to bring about the required changes or improvements in the involuntary—be it the kidney, liver, spleen, heart or lungs.

He was called names like 'hard', 'angry', 'hot-tempered'; he was anything but. He was loving, kind, compassionate like none other. He wanted yoga to reach everyone; he envisioned the world reaping the benefits of this beautiful, ancient art, which is also a practical science. Young or old, man or woman, rich or poor, he wanted yoga to spread deep into the heart of every person who came to learn. He was tough on lethargy and indiscipline, never on his students, and it takes an artiste to walk that thin line.

He never distracted his students with promises of meditative states, better spiritual evolution than others, etc., but only promised them more work in the asana. And there is a huge audience for honesty—over 40 million students across the globe are willing to practice asanas in their pure form.

If this has been achieved, it is one man's work—Guruji B.K.S. Iyengar, who always said and maintained that the school of yoga is very different from the business of yoga.

Easy exercises/asana practice at home

1. Easy home exercises for senior citizens
2. Easy asana at home
3. The plank challenge

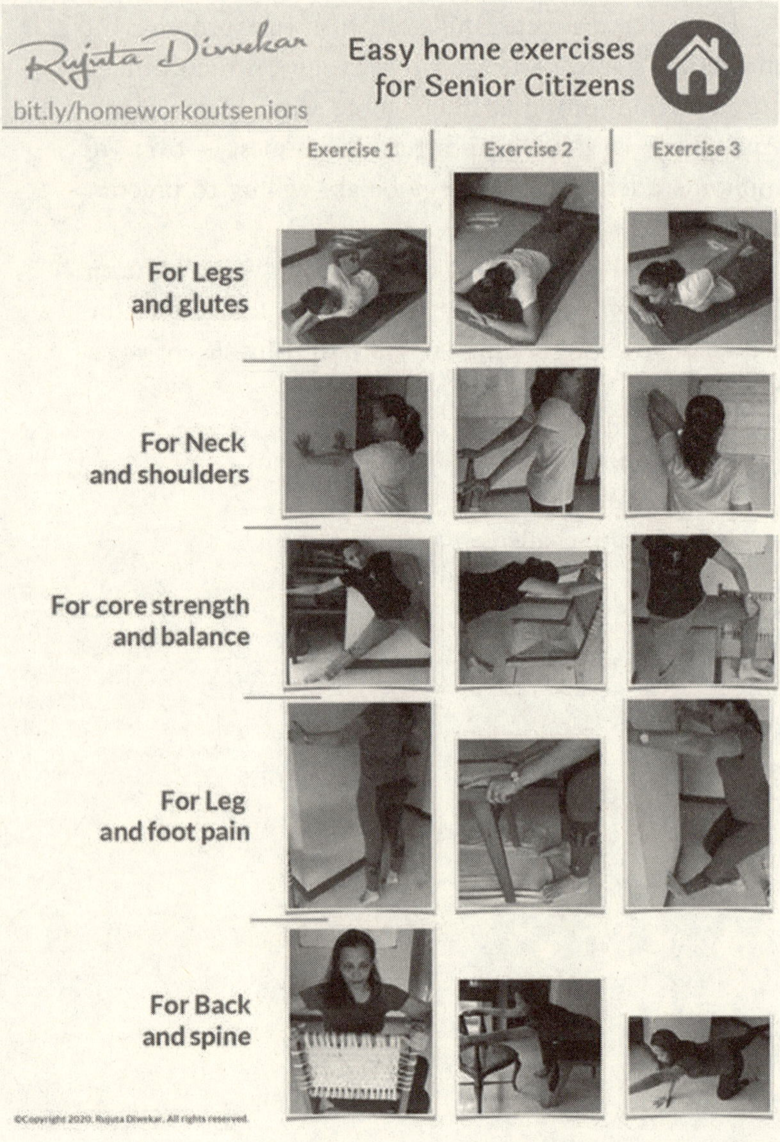
Rujuta Diwekar
bit.ly/homeworkoutseniors
Easy home exercises for Senior Citizens
Exercise 1
Exercise 2
Exercise 3
For Legs and glutes
For Neck and shoulders
For core strength and balance
For Leg and foot pain
For Back and spine
©Copyright 2020. Rujuta Diwekar. All rights reserved.

Easy Asana at home

Rujuta Diwekar

Videos - https://bit.ly/easyhomeasana

Asana for immunity	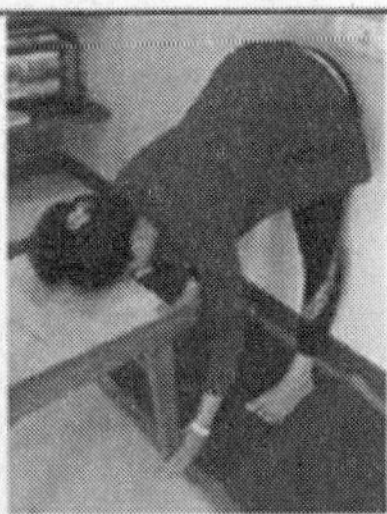	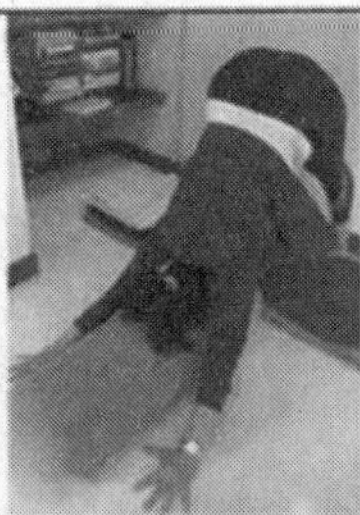	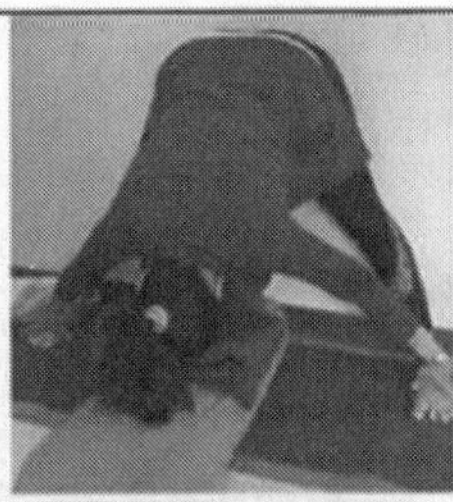
Asana for BP/ Stress/ Anxiety	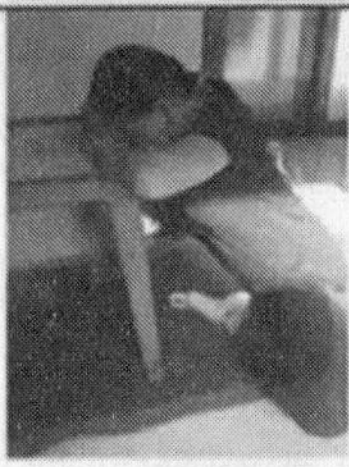	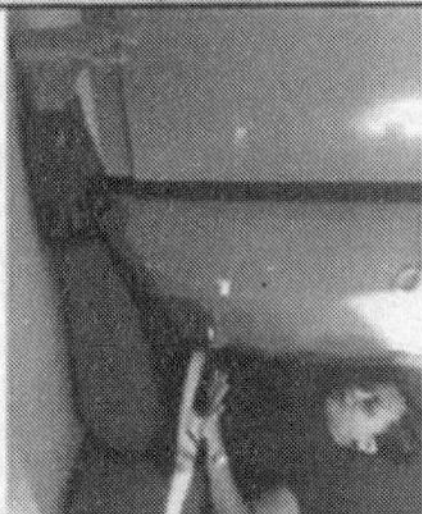	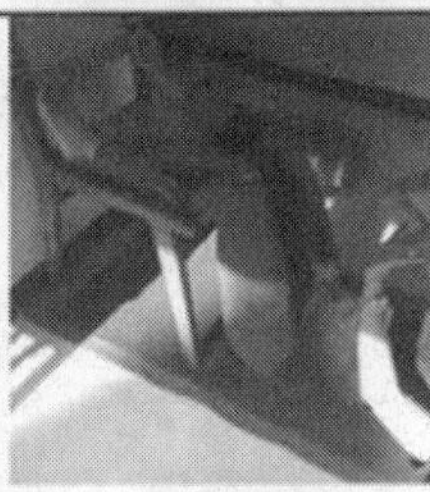
Asana for constipation	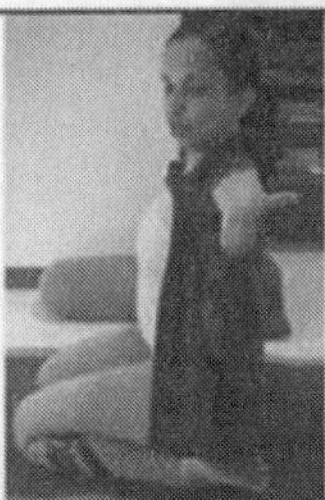	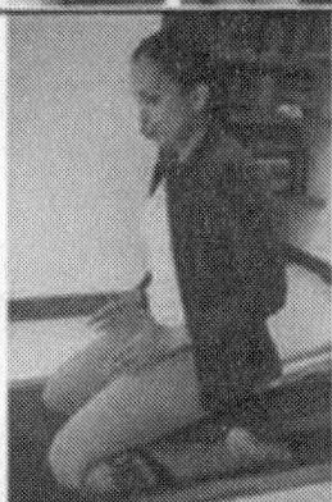	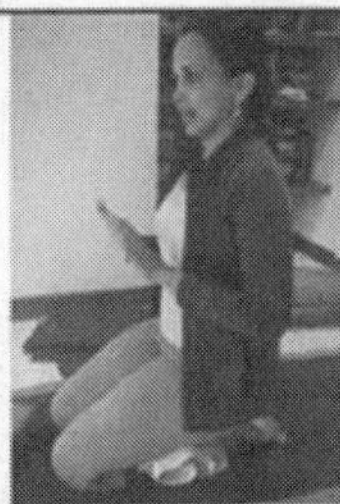
Asana for aches, pain and recovery	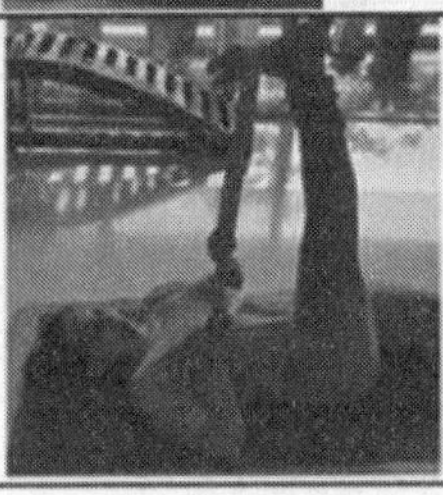	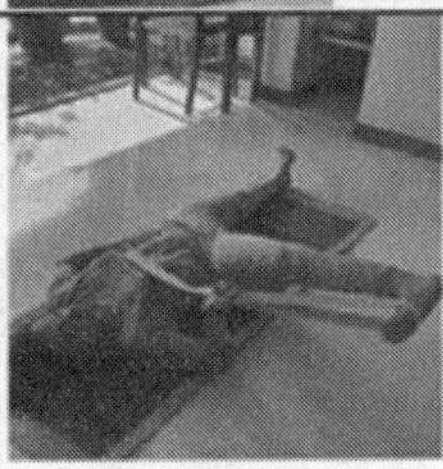	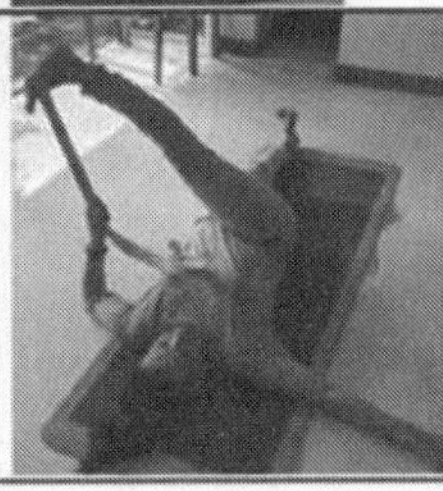

The plank challenge

'Home exercise and diet (HEAD)' project

Rujuta Diwekar

Start from a count of 5. Build to 60 and move to next level.

<table>
<tr><td>Level 1

Feet away from the wall

Body in one straight line</td><td>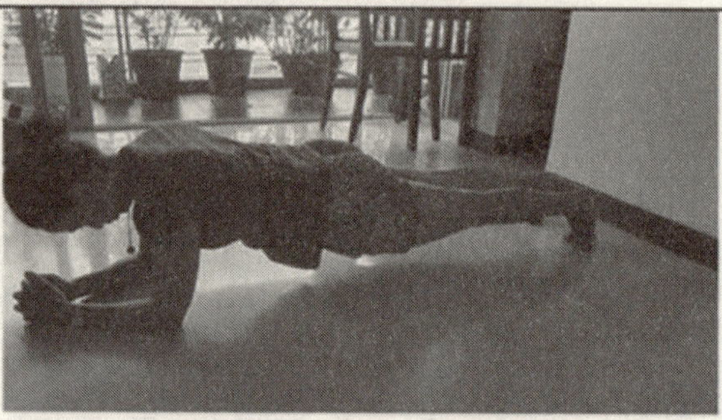</td></tr>
<tr><td>Level 2

Feet against the wall

Heel pressing on the wall</td><td>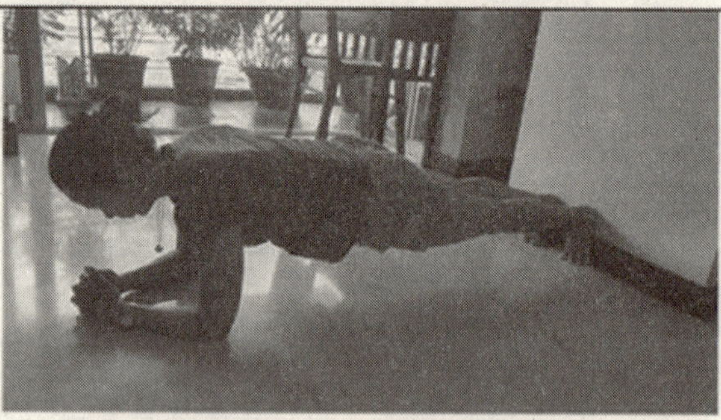</td></tr>
<tr><td>Level 3

Feet up the wall

Congrats!</td><td>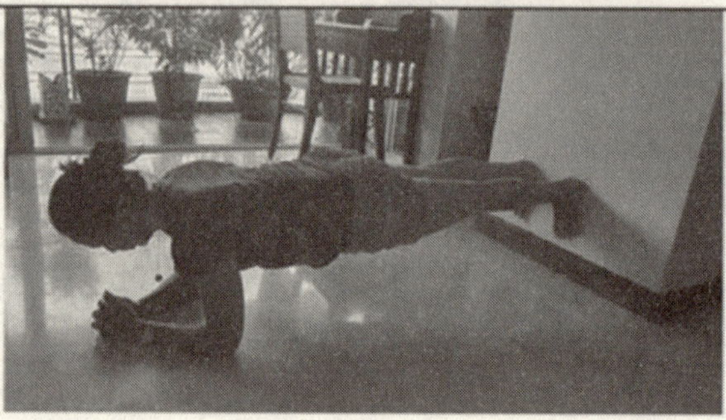</td></tr>
</table>

“

RUJUTA SAYS...

Our kids rather have smart brains and fast reflexes than smart phones with fast internet.

Our future—our children—and our past—the food traditions from our ancestors—makes our present such a gift!

When junk is the easy and convenient choice, the next gen gets fat.

If we indulge our children with attention, love and laughter, they will not need chips, chocolates, cupcakes for happiness.

Let’s raise our girls to be proud and not embarrassed of their success and our boys of their softness.

We owe it to our children to recognise junk food even if it comes with toys, fanfare or salads on the insides!

”

4B. KIDS' HEALTH

Our children are our true wealth, our future, and the ones who hold the key to our heart and to our hopes. Our young population is, however, not in its best shape. We are probably the only country with a high number of underweight children—at 43 per cent, the highest amongst developing countries—and also the second-highest number of obese children in the world. Double whammy, and then add the third angle to this, micronutrient deficiencies: anaemia, low levels of vitamin B12 and vitamin D, etc. It's a complex problem, one that will need urgent steps from multiple agencies and government bodies to get resolved, but in the meanwhile, there are things that we can change as parents, schools, and society. The big thing that needs to change is our attitude and awareness. We can then take small but significant steps towards ensuring a better future for our children, one that is filled with health and joy. A better today is the only way to have a better future.

Six ways to keep our children healthy

Here are the top six things we can adopt as a family/society to protect the interests of our future generations:

1. Say 'no'

i.Family was a five-year-long study across the European Union, that looked into the environment kids grow up in to understand rising obesity amongst EU adolescents.

Here's the message that they have for parents: Say No. The next time your kids pull out their pester power over an iPad, a box of chips, cola or chocolate, say a firm 'no'. It is, as the study reveals, the only way to protect your children from developing cardio-metabolic syndrome in the future. That includes obesity, diabetes, heart disease, fatty liver, etc.

2. Move

Fatty liver, or non-alcoholic fatty liver disease as it is called, is a reversible condition but it is affecting more kids than ever in the last five years. This happens when there is hyperinsulinemia, a condition where the muscles stop responding to insulin and the body produces more than required levels of this hormone, which the liver then has to deal with. Helping kids build age-appropriate muscle strength is important here and that comes from staying active and simply playing (real, not virtual).

3. Cook

Nutrition societies across the globe are of the opinion that children should be involved in cooking when they are as young as four years old and that it should be a part of the school syllabus. Cooking, after all, is a life-saving skill, and when our children learn how much water goes into atta before it turns into roti, or how a little teaspoon of dahi in lukewarm milk can turn into curd within eight hours, etc., their life takes a turn for the better and opens endless opportunities of creativity.

4. Decode advertisements

In South American countries like Chile, you cannot advertise packaged products to children, a far cry from our on-screen mommies who gush over their little one (always male) as he drinks corn syrup- and preservative-loaded powders in milk that are masked as protein and vitamin D sources or things that help improve memory or height. There is even a commercial now that lures kids into winning an iPhone after watching certain hours of a cartoon channel. Virat Kohli should get an award for refusing to endorse a cola giant anymore. But mostly, we don't hold our celebrities accountable; they can sell us cola, chips, instant noodles as long as there is a good-looking commercial with a hummable jingle to go with.

The food industry casts a wide net and ensures that you are always buying, not thinking or cooking. In a sense, we are truly cola-nised. In the absence of a regulation on commercials, the onus is on parents and schools to actively teach kids how to decode them.

5. Undo alcohol

There is nothing cool about introducing your sixteen-year-old or even your eighteen-year-old to alcohol. Instead, you need to introduce them to ways to prevent non-communicable diseases (NCDs) in the future and protect them from the suffering and disabilities they cause. Alcohol, along with tobacco, a poor diet and lack of exercise is one of the four major risk factors for NCDs. While we do acknowledge the other three as risks, alcohol has gotten away by projecting itself as cool and socially acceptable. This needs to change, and the media has a role to play. So does civil society.

6. Equality

Gender equations at home affect children's health in ways that we cannot fathom, but the effects are for all of us to see. When we go to villages and see little girls in uniforms washing clothes after school and little boys playing cricket in the field, we must know that we play out a version of this in our homes too.

The father switches between television channels, rarely cooks and stares at his gadget at the family table, while the mother stays responsible and is on her toes for daily household chores. This is a far cry from the gender-equal society that we hope our children grow up in. Recognise this and change this, now.

Don't eat your hearts out!

'You can come out and eat, i told her.' That was my client, twenty-two-year-old Asha, talking about her nine-year-old cousin, who lived with her as part of the large joint family. As Asha's eyes welled up, i, too, found myself looking down, trying not to get emotional about the story of this child who dared not eat freely in front of other people. It had all started, Asha said, when the child began to develop a bit of a tummy. Seeing her changed body, her parents began to have nightmares about how excess weight would spell doom for, hold your breath, their marriage plans for her. All this was, of course, communicated to the child, whose food intake was now restricted. So she began to hide and eat every time she wanted to have a snack or needed to eat a little more regular food than what had been apportioned to her. She ate in the loo, the doll's house, under the bed, any place far away from the prying eyes of her mum and maids. It's shameful that we, as parents, don't guide our kids into puberty with the information and compassion they need. Developing a rounded stomach around the time of puberty is a natural developmental change, and a desirable one. What is undesirable is imposing food bans on growing children, and not providing them with access to open spaces and sports, which would help them deal in a positive way with these changes. Hearing such stories convinces me how important it is for parents to educate themselves about the basics of eating right, keeping fit, sleeping on time and helping their children nurture healthy relationships with their own bodies. No one should have to hide and eat, least of all our daughters. Daughters who hide and eat turn into daughters who hide and puke three or four years later, and spend a lifetime fighting with their bodies.

Childhood obesity and parenting—FAQs

Q. What can parents do/not do to inculcate healthy eating habits amongst children from a young age?

First of all, you have to acknowledge that you are raising kids in 2020 and it's tough being both a child and a parent in the age of information and technology overload. The best way to put a child off healthy eating habits is to talk carb, protein, fat, calories, etc. on the dining table. It makes eating a chore and makes them feel inadequate.

Mealtimes should be what they are meant to be—a time for everyone to be together and enjoy good food and have a good time. Food should be spoken about in terms of culture, climate, crop cycle and not food groups. This allows children to see food and eating as a natural, social act and encourages them to eat responsibly. The key here is to not just talk but do; kids watch more than they listen.

Parents should also monitor their own eating habits better and work at building a long-term and sustainable healthy lifestyle. i have often noticed that parents who have a poor body image invariably superimpose that on their kids too. Being on extreme weight-loss diets—only protein, only salads, etc.—or an obsession with exercise often compounds the problem. 'i really need to knock off five pounds' may seem like a harmless thing to say around a child, but it lays the foundation to a twisted relationship with body weight, about fitting in and health in general.

Q. Outside of home, is the easy availability of junk food, soft drinks, etc. leading to a dramatic increase in childhood obesity? Are there any other factors to be considered?

The whole food environment needs to change. Making it about junk food or soft drinks is like blaming the child for not having enough will power to eat right or exercise, but the fact remains that we are raising them in an obesogenic environment. Some examples are:

- Poor planning of cities and towns, not having access to footpaths or cycling tracks to go to school.
- Buildings having more parking spaces than open spaces to play.
- Easy availability of junk food around and inside schools.

• Inaction of government in preventing the vulnerable age group from being targeted by food advertising and marketing.

Q. Will setting strict rules when it comes to consuming junk food, etc. have a long-term impact on the eating habits of kids?

No. The fact is that they are going to grow up and then you will be at the receiving end of teenage rebellion. Instead, educate them about how junk food is a global industry and how the same food is in every mall, every airport, etc. Tell them how selling toys with junk food is banned in some countries, Chile for example, but not in ours. Teach them about how the food industry is often not responsible or ethical about garbage they produce. Get them to carry a bottle and fill it at the airport instead of just picking bottled water in the aircraft. It's not about avoiding calories but living more responsibly and sensibly. It's okay if they have junk sometimes; the idea is that they have to be able to identify it as junk and not associate either aspiration or prestige with it.

If a celeb is endorsing junk, teach your child that they are getting paid to pose, drink and eat that food on camera. Children are quick to adopt lifestyle changes when they see food from a broader angle, and are especially sensitive to both the economic and ecological aspects of food. Make the conversation wholesome—if you talk from a point of view of sugar or calories or fat, there will be a sugar/calorie/fat-free version of the same junk, and you will be left fighting a lost battle.

Top three myths on child nutrition

Myth 1: It's okay to let them watch TV or the iPad if it helps them finish a meal.

Fact: It's important to teach them to eat with all their senses and not mindlessly. Eating while viewing means bigger bites, faster speed of consumption and eventually digestion issues and higher risk of non-communicable diseases. The EU's i.Family study also links TV viewing while eating to higher demand for sugar-sweetened beverages (colas, etc.) and junk food from kids.

Myth 2: They must be about the same height and weight as their peers or cousins.

Fact: Each child has their own unique growth curve, and as long as they are active and alert in school and regularly play/participate in sports, their height and weight is not a concern.

Myth 3: They must eat sabzis or salads to get vitamins, dals for protein and milk for calcium.

Fact: There is no one source for one nutrient. The idea is to eat a more diverse diet that is local, seasonal and traditional, and to complement it with playing outdoors and a regular bedtime. It is only when the basics are in place that the body is capable of assimilating all nutrients including protein, calcium and vitamins.

A note for all girls who just finished taking their 10th or 12th standard exams

1. Run, play and walk around, there will be plenty of time to sit in cafes later.

Builds better bones, stronger spines and ensures pain-free periods for the rest of your life.

2. Drink kokum sherbet, aam panha and bel sherbet; there will be plenty of time to sip cola later.

Promotes growth of healthy bacteria, nurtures intestinal mucosa and ensures flawless skin for the rest of your life.

3. Go to bed by 10.30 p.m. every night; there will be plenty of time to party all night later.

Regulates your hormones, keeps them in a state of balance and ensures that the brain works at its optimum for the rest of your life.

Three easy ways to teach your child to spot food that is bad for them

1. Comes with a cartoon character on the packaging.
2. Comes with a free (often single-use plastic) toy.
3. Comes with a contest that offers to send you abroad or give you an iPad, etc.

Basically, if there's an ad, it's bad.

Top six tips that every parent can follow for kids' health

1. Gadget-free meals.
2. Say NO to pester power.
3. Active holidays together.
4. Internet fasting once a month.
5. Farm over a mall.
6. Speak in the local language.

Five ideas for school snacks for your kids

1. Roti with jaggery and ghee is rich in iron and minerals and a quick go-to snack for the long ride back home or post a sports class.
2. Homemade laddoos made with aliv (garden cress seeds), jaggery and coconut ensure that moods don't swing and energy levels don't drop.
3. Banana is great even on days your child feels like skipping lunch in school. It contains enough nutrients to equip them for the long day.
4. Nimbu sherbet with a little ginger, kesar and black pepper is great for the stomach and works as an antidote to the indigestion and fatigue that dehydration causes.
5. Homemade chakli, mathri and chivda are healthy options that leave your children well-nourished for all their daily tasks.

Five rules for happy and healthy kids

1. Wake up and eat nuts, never go to school hungry.
2. Carry a steel dabba with a homemade snack—no plastic containers or bottles for kids, especially when pre-pubescent.
3. Roti or bhakri with jaggery and ghee once every day—especially when the season changes—to stay strong and resistant to infections and flus.
4. Celebrations are best enjoyed in open spaces by running at crazy speeds on your own two feet. Not by sitting down in restaurants and stuffing your mouth with junk.

5. Limit screen time to max thirty minutes per day. More than that will interfere with how tall, strong and fast you can get.

Tips for kids and teens during home-school

1. Have a homemade nashta of poha or upma or idli or dosa or paratha or thalipeeth or thepla + fresh fruit, either as a meal by itself or along with breakfast (rich in vitamin A, vitamin B and polyphenols—aids digestion and is a mood enhancer; also reduces craving for junk food).
2. Legumes and rice for lunch—chana or rajma or chole or moong or matki or any local legume, soaked overnight and cooked well the next day and served with rice. End with a glass of homemade chaas (combination of pre and pro biotic; mineral- and amino acid-rich meal that is also easy to digest).
3. Bowl of dahi set with black raisins—anytime in the day. Rich in B12 and iron, beats the heat and lethargy, improves hormonal health. Regulates appetite.
4. Early dinner—by 7 p.m. Paneer paratha, poori-sabzi, roti-sabzi roll, ajwain paratha, jowar or nachni bhakri with aloo bhaji, veg pulao with raita and homemade deep-fried papad. (Wholesome meals that are fun and kind of one dish; complete the nutrition profile and involve kids in planning and cooking.) Once a week—homemade pizza, pasta, pav bhaji or anything you fancy, but not later than 7 p.m.
5. Haldi-doodh or mango milkshake or gulkand-milk or fresh mango or banana around bedtime if hungry.

Special tip—five habits for good health:
i. No packaged cereals, cookies or chocolates.
ii. Regulated screen time.
iii. Once a week, family movie night.
iv. Daily play of sixty to ninety minutes + six suryanamaskars.
v. Help out with household chores every day—at least thirty minutes (age-appropriate and safe, supervise as needed).

Kids health and government policies

Here is a shortlist of what governments can and must do for public health/kids' health.

1. If governments do want to encourage us to eat healthy, then they should first enact laws regarding pricing, promotion and placement of ultra-processed food products or junk foods. You really don't need the government to tell you that a burger is not healthy, but you need government intervention to ensure that the burger company doesn't go after your children with toys, ads and glitzy marketing.
2. Push for local food systems to get more resilient. The Andhra government's move to launch zero-budget natural farming to 6 million farmers in 8 million hectares by 2024 is a commendable and much-needed step in the right direction. It will ensure that native crops get a boost, intercropping (growing more on the same land) thrives, water wastage is reduced and will greatly reduce the use of chemical pesticides and fertilisers. If this is followed by

cleaning up the food environment where local vegetables and fruits are sold, it would be even better. Imagine walking into a mandi in a clean environment with your cloth bag in hand, talking to your sabzi wali about her child's 10th standard exams. Wait, it wasn't that long ago when we actually did this, till we lost our cities and souls in the aspiration of becoming the next Shanghai or Singapore.

3. Ensure that FSI for new buildings is not granted unless there is a compulsory open green space for children to play and for the elderly to walk. Restrictions on number of cars bought or parked per flat can also be considered so that more space opens out for free movement in residential areas.

4. Make public parks more safe and accessible to adolescent and teenage girls. Currently, all our open spaces are dominated by boys; maybe consider a reservation for a few days every month if not every week?

5. Include farming and agriculture as a compulsory part of primary education. The current curriculum of health advisors, be it doctors or dietitians, don't even make a passing reference to land use, farming or regional/local foods. At least start with updating existing food and nutrition syllabi?

IPL and kids' obesity

The nine-year-old who lives upstairs met me in the lift. 'Wow,' i said, looking at his kit. 'Where do you play?' 'Khar gym.' 'What are you good at?' After due consideration he says, 'Hmm, batting i am so-so, wicket-keeping i am okay, bowling i am really good at.' 'Wow,' i said, louder this time and we high-fived. Yeah, IPL is here and everyone who is anyone is playing. The camera pans to the kids in the stands. 'It's just so heartening to see so many children out there, supporting the game...' say the commentators at least once during the four-hour game.

The thing is, IPL is here to stay; it's beautiful, young and glamorous. It's changed the way we view and consume all things sports, from cricket to kabbadi, putting sport straight into the bracket of aspirational. There's money, fame and a million followers on social media, it's all very heady. The sheer visibility has been milked by everyone from protestors to sponsors and, as Sunil Gavaskar puts it, IPL is a soft target. And so i am talking about an even softer target, the children who watch the game. And how the ultra-processed food, commonly called junk food, which sponsors ad breaks, franchises and even cheerleading squads may affect them.

The reason being that Indian kids are getting fat at an alarming rate. We may land up having 17 million obese kids by 2025. Obviously, we ought to protect our children, as obesity is the leading cause of non-communicable diseases like cancer, hypertension, diabetes, and also a leading cause of early death, poor quality of life and impaired childhood experience. Nutrition academicians and social lobbying across the globe are asking businesses, the food industry specifically, to respond more ethically to this global epidemic. Mexico led the way with its sugar tax, Chile has responded with food labels that allow kids to identify junk food and has banned the sale of toys along with junk food, the US is debating the reduction of serving sizes and we, well ...

Recently, there was an interesting study published about sports sponsorships and how they promote junk food to children. While this was a US-based study, the scene is not very different in India. While sport sends out a positive message about health and fitness, the strong visibility of junk food during games sends out a confusing message, to say the least. Eating right and avoiding junk food is one of the basic steps of staying healthy, one that every kid easily understands. What they don't understand is, what is a burger logo doing on the jersey of their fav team. What we don't understand (fully) as parents is how this leads to cued eating in a child—the demand for more junk food, tantrums over it or hunger for it even when their stomach is already full. Or, in general, a positive correlation between junk food and sporting greatness. This even extends to casual conversations of burning off calories the next day (in older adolescents and even adults), and the flawed belief that exercise can repair a poor diet. It doesn't. Poor dietary habits come with the big cost of obesity and NCDs and the poor are more vulnerable to it than the rich.

A little bit of self-regulation from the franchises will go a long way in helping our kids, especially those from the weaker sections of society, to stay away/have limited exposure to junk food. Of all the cricket tournaments, the kids and youth segment watch IPL the most. Advertisers know this and they also know that they are watching this with both parents (IPL has a large female viewership too), and this co-viewing allows kids the opportunity to influence the decisions of parents. So you will find even non-food ads with kids—the idea is to use them to influence the decision-makers and the money-spenders, the parents. So, i am also calling for a bit of self-regulation from the advertising industry, especially when it comes to marketing junk food to children. i checked out the Advertising Council of India's website, and while there is a general code for self-regulation, i didn't find one specifically for children. In other countries, you have one, and that ad where the wink girl tells you to eat that chocolate and win that wristband would be found to have flouted it. So would that dad who says, want this cola, accept my friendship request.

The fact is that we are living in an obesogenic environment, and it will need a multipronged approach—more open, greener spaces, footpaths for kids to safely walk to and walk back from school/colleges, changes in pricing and policies by the government agencies (not allowing Rs 5 chips and junk food packets to be sold for example), regulating the number of junk food ads kids watch on TV channels (like Jamie Oliver's recent #adenough campaign), etc. But not signing on a junk food company as a team sponsor is low hanging fruit that IPL franchises should seriously consider. It makes for good PR, CSR and even helps improve credibility of teams who otherwise pledge to do their bit for the underprivileged.

As parents, we should help our children understand celebrity endorsements and team sponsorships. Very plainly, we need to tell children that your fav cricketer is eating it on screen because he is getting paid for it. Or your fav team's jersey which you can buy from their website has a junk food logo because they get paid to place it there. This is business; teach them to separate it from health. And as parents, if you must ask for more accountability, it should be from the food industry, franchise owners and government agencies (and not specifically in that order); celebs are small fry here. For all of Virat Kohli's sporting greatness and personal decision to not make many crores by renewing the contract with Pepsi (in a world where a cola ad is the ultimate marker of success, this is nothing short of a revolutionary step), when his team, RCB, endorses a pizza, it lands on his jersey.

Overall, what we need to understand is that childhood obesity is a ticking bomb, one that needs urgent intervention. Here's calling on all franchisee owners to take the captain's lead and do their bit for the loyal and vulnerable customer base, the kids, and ensure that IPL fever does not turn into an illness.

RUJUTA SAYS...

To all women who wake up tired, the only cure for fatigue is rest, not caffeine, exercise, or guilt.

The ability to hold on to yourself no matter how stretched you feel is called strength. And that is just one good reason why every working woman must exercise.

To me, an empowered woman is the one who feels happy and not guilty when she eats something she likes.

A well-raised girl is always kind, patient and forgiving—towards herself.

Every time you look in the mirror, smile, it's the best (and cheapest) anti-ageing tool on earth. :=)

Strong and sundar women come in every size and shape! What makes them beautiful is that they carry their own weight. :-)

4C. WOMEN

My advice to women of all age groups

Teenagers: Never go on a diet.
Twenties: Don't just get skinny for your wedding day, focus on eating right every day.
Thirties: Your bone mineral density peaks, time to do more with your body.
Forties: Be comfortable in your body, don't succumb to ageism.
Fifties: It's important to have a daily routine.
Sixties: Enjoy all new roles and continue to follow your dreams.
Seventies and above: Share your wisdom while continuing to take care of yourself.

The fat girl complex

Most women that i work with think of themselves as too fat and too big. Interestingly, this has nothing to do with their size, shape or weight. So a twenty-five-year-old who is 54 kg will tell me that she's so fat that she can't bear to look at herself. A forty-year-old who's 69 kg will say the same thing about herself, and so will a sixty-five-year-old who's 85 kg.

Over the years, what i have realised is that 'fat' is more a state of mind than of the body. And that whether we are twenty-five/fifty-five years old, or 54/86 kg, what matters to our health and fitness is how we treat ourselves. How we see ourselves.

What i promise you is that women who see themselves as productive individuals who are worthy of food, get fitter and leaner with time. On the other hand, those who see themselves as fat at twenty-five, only seem to get fatter at fifty-five. Only this time, with more illnesses and poorer self-esteem thanks to all the dieting and deprivation in between.

The fastest way to lose weight is to be grateful for your body, to love it and accept it unconditionally. To buy clothes that you would love to wear without any hang-ups about size. Health is not a number, it is a state of mind. And we are fine at every size.

The next time you see yourself in a mirror, tell yourself how wow you look.

Women and the health connection

Time and again, the one thing that i have seen in my career is disregard and indifference towards our indigenous food wisdom and native cuisines. And mostly it is because the bearers, upholders and practitioners of that are women.

Take the example of haldi. Traditional diets made intelligent and liberal use of haldi—from tadkas of sabzis and dals to cups of haldi milk. But then, in comes diet advice and sabzis get replaced with steamed veggies or raw salads. While we search for health in deprivation, we miss out on the obvious.

We also miss out on the fact that the advice masquerading as 'science' is actually about economics. What it does is that it takes the control away from a large number of individual women and puts it in the hands of a few big companies and professionals. And while you seek glory in deprivation, they are busy making money by selling you the exact same ingredient that they first very 'scientifically' and systematically removed from your diet. So haldi is now in curcumin pills or shots. Ghee is in bullet coffee. And singdana is peanut butter.

Anyways, women, mostly belonging to East Indian or agri communities, pound the fresh haldi. They toil in the sun as they crush the haldi or make bottle masala for you. The whole area is filled with the aroma and the sound of their bangles. They sometimes hum a song or tell you a story that will touch a chord. And that's when you realise that health is all-encompassing, it is not shape or size, it is people and their wellbeing. Especially of those who are without a voice, the women.

Women's diet and effect on children

Women of reproductive age, fifteen to forty-nine years (our primary healthcare-givers), often fall short of eating a diverse diet—grains, legumes, seeds, dairy, fruits, veggies, etc. (called minimum dietary diversity for women—MDD-W). This leads to low dietary diversity for infants and children too, resulting in micronutrient deficiencies like anaemia, low levels of vitamin B12, vitamin D, poor immune function and lack of optimum growth milestones.

It's easy to stay healthy and achieve dietary diversity if we learn to eat according to what grows locally, what changes seasonally and if we learn to cook and eat first (and not always after kids, husband).

Here's to women breaking the shackles of calorie counting and weight loss, so that our daughters stay on top, well-nurtured and capable of leading a bloody good life.

Why every woman after forty should learn inversions

When we turn forty, we often wonder if we must do something special or different to ensure that we don't prematurely age.

Here's an interesting take that one of my Iyengar yoga teachers, Karin O'Bannon, had on it. According to her, all women must practice inversions daily after they turn forty. Because most times, as women approach forty, they realise that they have spent a lifetime being good, obedient girls, but in the process, may have lost out on their true selves. This, according to her, even reflected in their asana practice—being good with forward bends but fearful of inversions. Fearful of using their own inner strength (core strength) to hold themselves up against convention or conditioning (gravity, in this case).

However, Iyengar yoga has multiple ways to learn inversions, a step at a time. It might not give you the instant thrill of an upside-down, but teaches you how to engage which muscle. That way, when you go against the norm or gravity, you are still safe, secure and graceful.

Note: Of course, you don't have to wait till you turn forty. The earlier you learn inversions, the better it is.

Body weight, size and happiness

i decided to describe a picture of real-life beautiful women and list down their qualities so that we realise that beauty cannot be captured or conceptualised by size or weight, it cannot be grasped with the camera and, more importantly, like love, we often stumble upon it when we are not searching for it.

So here are the qualities:

1. Busy—doing their bit in their lives so they really have no time to pose, click multiple pix and fuss over which is the best one to go on FB.
2. Bright—run their own errands and time it well so that they can do an evening walk while buying milk or sabzi. In every aspect of life, optimise the ek teer do nishaan policy.
3. Bindaas—eco-aware and not self-conscious. Carry a dabba to buy daily milk and avoid use of plastic, doesn't matter if anyone thinks you are a bhenji types. In the same vein, wear anything you want, anyway you want, with jacket, without, dupatta over shoulder/head, anything at all—your life, your bloody choice.
4. Bantaai—cultivate a gang of girls (outside of work and family) who will walk the path with them, whether it's for a walk, errands, coffee or just for laughs.

Beautiful at every size and shape

Having a body weight number as the 'target' or 'aim' that one must achieve is one of the many ways in which women disrespect themselves and their intelligence on a daily basis. Endless data is available in medical, fitness and nutrition journals to show beyond reasonable doubt that health is not guaranteed by a certain—read, low—body weight. So this weight-loss obsession, something that people like me live off literally, is not about health, it's about, well sorry to say, looking like a boy or, at best, like a pre-pubescent girl. It's about feeling good one may argue, but then what has that got to do with a number?

What makes us feel good is how well we treat ourselves, and that includes whether or not we take the time and effort to nourish ourselves. i have seen women go through near-death experiences to 'achieve', however short-lived, a certain size and body weight. Surgical procedures, starvation diets, mindless exercise, you name it. And funny as it may seem, in all my years of working, i haven't met a single man who has said to me that if he lost 5 or 15 kg then he would be taken more seriously. Women somehow do seem to chase size or weight for self-respect, love and acceptance. But it's like this—money can't buy you happiness and body weight can't give you self-worth either.

i think of food and fitness as things that empower us women to be ourselves, chase our dreams and speak our minds. A number of women i work with have told me that even after the soup/salad starvation routine to reach an impossibly low body weight or size, they felt anything but good, forget great; mostly they felt weak and dead. Food makes both our physical bodies and our minds, say our ancient sciences and practical philosophies of yoga and Ayurveda. The food we eat should fill both our mind and body with energy, enthusiasm and optimism. Counting calories, avoiding carbs, increasing the protein, is hardly a way to achieve that. Mostly because 'nutrition science' is still evolving, taking baby steps towards understanding how food consumption affects absorption, assimilation and excretion and how all this in turn affects health and wellbeing. That's exactly why what they called a villain yesterday, saturated fat for example, is the hero today.

The food and the weight-loss industry, on the other hand, looks at us women as their target consumers. The more we reduce our life and its goals and purpose to fitting into a size 6 before the new year let's say, the more they thrive. They thrive on our confusion, conflicting expert opinions and media images/advertisements. Recently, an Australian swimming champion was reduced to size 4, from her original 8, in pictures where she endorsed a brand of swimwear. Thankfully, she didn't find herself 'pretty' in the photos and asked to be 'plumped' back to original size. The message is the same: if you are not a certain size, that medal win, or anything else, is less valuable or preferably has no meaning.

Our home-bred food wisdom is not keen on reducing us to numbers or sizes. Thankfully, we are still a country where grandmothers prod us to eat all the good food—the mithai during celebrations, the ghee, coconut, rice, milk, the bhakris with sabzis made with heritage recipes, bringing us an unbroken chain of love, wisdom, nourishment shared by the women across generations. It's important that we don't turn our back on it, it's important that we don't see it as evil or damaging just because it's 'high calorie'. It's important that we nourish our bodies and don't turn away from love, even when it comes in the form of food. And, more importantly, we must pass this to the next generation of women.

It's important to remember that a woman who is herself is the one who is going to turn heads in a room packed with poor copies of each other. It's the woman who chases her dreams fearlessly who is celebrated and accepted, first by herself and then society. That a woman's job in life is to listen to the voice inside her head, not to her husband/son/father in whatever order. Borrowing from the movie *The Help*, 'You is smart ... you is beautiful ... you is important'. Yes, at every body weight and size.

THIS IS WHAT NUTRITION SCIENCE AND LATEST RESEARCH SAYS ABOUT WEIGHT LOSS

1. 25–30 per cent of obese people are metabolically healthy, i.e. their blood sugars, cholesterol, etc., are well regulated. However, when people lose weight quickly through dieting, not only do they gain the weight back, but now they are no longer metabolically healthy. They are at a 150 per cent higher risk of diabetes, heart disease, cancer, etc. A good indicator of unhealthy weight loss is if you lose too much weight from the thigh area (very thin legs). Losing about 5–10 per cent of your total weight in a year is considered healthy and sustainable.

2. Losing weight through unsustainable diets, fasting, etc., especially when you are already metabolically weak, i.e. suffering from diabetes, cancer, etc., is that much more harmful.

3. Meal frequency is positively linked to healthy weight loss. Regular meals throughout the day lead to better metabolic health and sustainable weight loss in the long term. Especially important is to have an early breakfast (before 9 a.m.) and an early lunch (before 2 p.m.).

4. Maintaining gut bacteria diversity is crucial for overall health and weight loss. A meal with a combination of probiotics + prebiotics, along with short chain fatty acids (SCFA), is the ideal meal to increase satiety, reduce inflammation, prevent infections and maintain intestinal integrity. In other

words, traditional Indian meals, like dal-chawal-ghee or khichdi with dahi, pickle, etc., are perfectly suited for gut health and healthy weight loss.

5. Governments and policy makers should make 'food based' diet guidelines and not 'nutrient based', so that the general public doesn't get confused between carbs/fats/proteins and instead finds health and joy in eating local, seasonal, traditional foods.

The overall message:

• Losing weight is not important, metabolic health is the key.

• Dieting leads to increased risk of cancer, diabetes, etc.

• Follow traditional diet patterns and don't decide food based on carbs/protein/fat.

(Highlights from the 2019 European nutrition conference in Dublin, Ireland.)

INDEX